Biological Functions of Carbohydrates

TERTIARY LEVEL BIOLOGY

A series covering selected areas of biology at advanced undergraduate level. While designed specifically for course options at this level within Universities and Polytechnics, the series will be of great value to specialists and research workers in other fields who require a knowledge of the essentials of a subject.

Titles in the series:

Experimentation in Biology	Ridgman
Methods in Experimental Biology	Ralph
Visceral Muscle	Huddart and Hunt
Biological Membranes	Harrison and Lunt
Comparative Immunobiology	Manning and Turner
Water and Plants	Meidner and Sheriff
Biology of Nematodes	Croll and Matthews
An Introduction to Biological Rhythms	Saunders
Biology of Ageing	Lamb
Biology of Reproduction	Hogarth
An Introduction to Marine Science	Meadows and Campbell
Biology of Fresh Waters	Maitland
An Introduction to Developmental Biology	Ede
Physiology of Parasites	Chappell
Neurosecretion	Maddrell and Nordmann
Biology of Communication	Lewis and Gower
Population Genetics	Gale
Biochemistry and Structure of Cell Organelles	Reid and Leech
Developmental Microbiology	Peberdy
The Genetics of Microbes	Bainbridge
Endocrinology	Goldsworthy, Robinson and Mordue

TERTIARY LEVEL BIOLOGY

Biological Functions of Carbohydrates

DAVID J. CANDY, B.Sc., Ph.D.

Lecturer in Biochemistry
University of Birmingham

A HALSTED PRESS BOOK

John Wiley and Sons
New York—Toronto

Blackie & Son Limited
Bishopbriggs
Glasgow G64 2NZ

Furnival House
14–18 High Holborn
London WC1V 6BX

Published in the U.S.A. and Canada by
Halsted Press,
a Division of John Wiley and Sons Inc.,
New York

Library of Congress Cataloging in Publication Data

Candy, David John, 1936–
    Biological functions of carbohydrates.

    (Tertiary level biology)
    "A Halsted Press book."
    Bibliography: p.
    Includes index.
    1. Carbohydrate metabolism. 2. Carbohydrate in
the body. I. Title. [DNLM: 1. Carbohydrates—
Physiology. QU75 C219b]
QP701.C28   574.19'248   80-18668
ISBN 0-470-27038-1

Filmset by Advanced Filmsetters (Glasgow) Ltd.
Printed by Thomson Litho Ltd., East Kilbride, Scotland

Preface

The study of carbohydrates in biology is one of the longest-established aspects of the subject. In consequence, it is treated in most textbooks of biology and biochemistry—at least at an elementary level. However, certain areas of carbohydrate biochemistry have expanded rapidly over the past few years as a result of intense research activity. Such advances make this an opportune time to draw together the newer ideas of carbohydrate functions and to present them within a framework of established knowledge.

This book describes the role of carbohydrates in biology at a level which is suitable for undergraduate students in biochemistry, biology and the medical sciences. The subject is treated to the final-year level although, inevitably, advanced students will wish to expand their knowledge of particular topics by use of the reading list provided as an appendix.

Two areas are particularly emphasized. The first is the metabolic reactions of carbohydrates and the functions of such reactions in the organism. Here the regulation of metabolism in response to different physiological requirements is stressed, and concepts of compartmentation and transport are explored. The second area is concerned with the metabolism and functions of carbohydrate polymers. Here there has been a rapid expansion of research, particularly into the role of specific interactions of carbohydrates which occur, for example, at cell surfaces.

To illustrate these ideas, specific examples have been drawn from a number of different animals, plants and microorganisms. By selecting the appropriate organism as an experimental subject, the biologist can often demonstrate a phenomenon which has general applicability. This book reflects some of the wide range of organisms that have been used experimentally. Consideration has also been given to relationships be-

51785

tween defects in carbohydrate metabolism and disease in man, as observation of this type have frequently helped in our understanding of carbohydrate functions in the normal individual.

I wish to record my thanks to Dr. N. J. Kuhn who scrutinized the manuscript and made many invaluable suggestions. Helpful comments were also made by a number of colleagues, including Professor D. G. Walker, Dr. D. E. Briggs and Dr. A. P. Brown. Particular thanks are due also to Mrs. P. Hill for extensive assistance with the diagrams.

D.J.C.

Contents

CHAPTER ONE

CHEMISTRY OF CARBOHYDRATES

The term *carbohydrate* means literally "hydrate of carbon". Many simple carbohydrates (such as glucose) contain carbon, hydrogen and oxygen in the ratios implied by this name, and can be described by the empirical formula $(CH_2O)_n$. Such compounds have three or more carbon atoms, one of which bears a carbonyl group and the others hydroxyl groups.

There are, in addition, many other carbohydrates which do not fit the above description exactly but which are chemically related to the simple sugars. Such compounds may be derived from sugars by oxidation or reduction of the carbonyl group, or by replacement of one of the hydroxyl groups by some other group.

Carbohydrates are classified into monosaccharides, oligosaccharides or polysaccharides. The *monosaccharides* are sugars (such as glucose) in which all of the carbon atoms are joined together by direct carbon-to-carbon bonds. Monosaccharides are further classified according to their main functional group (aldehyde or ketone) and their chain length. For example, aldohexoses have an aldehyde group and six carbon atoms, whereas ketopentoses have a ketone group and five carbon atoms.

In the oligosaccharides, two or more monosaccharides are joined together by glycosidic linkages (p. 15) which have carbon–oxygen–carbon bonds linking the monosaccharide components. The oligosaccharides are subdivided into disaccharides, trisaccharides, tetrasaccharides, etc., which have two, three or four monosaccharide units respectively. The term *oligosaccharide* is generally taken to cover the range of from two to ten or so monosaccharide units per molecule. *Polysaccharides* are polymers containing more than about ten monosaccharides. Some polysaccharides

1

have a very large number of individual monosaccharide units per molecule, in some cases up to 500 000, giving molecular weights of nearly 100 million.

The monosaccharides

Isomerism

The atoms of sugars can be arranged in a number of different ways to give different isomeric forms, all of which have the same empirical formula. Thus the formula $C_6H_{12}O_6$ represents several different sugars including glucose, mannose and galactose. These sugars are *stereoisomers* of each other.

Stereoisomerism occurs in any organic compound in which a carbon

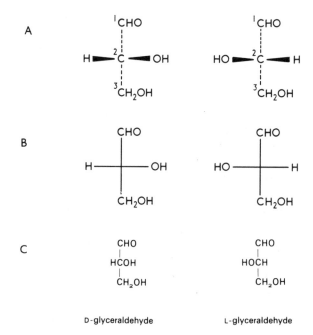

D-glyceraldehyde   L-glyceraldehyde

Figure 1.1 Stereoisomerism. In (A) the perspective formulae for the two isomers of glyceraldehyde show the tetrahedral arrangement of four substituents around the central carbon atom. The substituents in the two formulae have a different arrangement in space and are mirror images of each other. In the projection formulae (B) the convention is that horizontal substituents always project forwards and vertical substituents project backwards. These formulae can also be represented as shown in (C).

atom is substituted with four different atoms or groups. The groups can be arranged around the carbon in one of two ways such that one form is the mirror image of the other form, yet it is not possible to rotate either form so that it can be superimposed on the other (figure 1.1). Such isomeric forms have similar chemical properties to each other but rotate polarized light in opposite directions. The carbon atom in the centre of such a grouping is known as a *chiral* or *asymmetric* carbon, and the particular arrangement of groups around the carbon is known as the *configuration*.

The presence of stereoisomerism in a compound can be recognized by inspection of the structural formula to see whether any of the carbon atoms bears four different substituents. Figure 1.1 shows the structure of glyceraldehyde which is the simplest optically-active sugar. Carbon 2 of glyceraldehyde bears four different substituents (—CHO, —H, —OH, —CH$_2$OH) and is therefore chiral. The two isomers are known as D-glyceraldehyde (which rotates polarized light to the right) and L-glyceraldehyde (which rotates polarized light to the left).

The numbering system for monosaccharides is based on the location of the carbonyl group (or potential carbonyl group). The carbon atoms are numbered from one end of the chain such that the carbonyl group is given the lowest possible number. The formula is then written with carbon 1 at the top as shown for glyceraldehyde.

Stereoisomerism in many sugars is complicated by the presence of several different chiral carbons within the same molecule. Figure 1.2A shows the general structure of the aldohexose group of sugars. In the figure, the chiral carbons are marked with an asterisk, but their configurations are not specified. There are four such chiral carbons in the formula, and the configuration of each can be varied independently of the

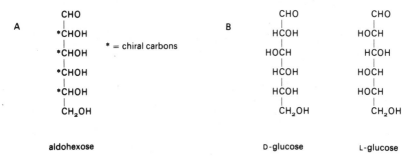

Figure 1.2 Formula A shows the general structure of aldohexoses in which the configuration of the chiral centres is not specified. In B the configuration of the chiral centres is shown for the two isomers of glucose.

others. The total number of possible isomers is 2^n, where n is the number of chiral carbons in the molecule. For the aldohexoses, the number of permutations is sixteen, of which eight are mirror images of the other eight. These two groups form members of the D- and L-series of sugars. Figure 1.2B shows the configurations for the D- and L- forms of glucose. Note that the configurations at *all* of the chiral carbons are different in the two different forms.

The convention for allocating a sugar to the D- or L-series depends on the configuration around the highest numbered carbon (the chiral carbon furthest from the main functional group). If the configuration at this carbon is the same as that of D-glyceraldehyde, with the hydroxyl group on the right-hand side, then the sugar belongs to the D-series. If the configuration at this centre is the same as for L-glyceraldehyde, the sugar belongs to the L-series, irrespective of the configuration at any of the other chiral centres. For glucose, the highest numbered chiral carbon is C5, and comparison of figure 1.2B with figure 1.1 shows that the configurations at this centre are the same as those of the corresponding isomers of glyceraldehyde..

The optical rotation of a sugar with more than one chiral carbon depends on contributions from the rotations of each optically active centre. Since these individual rotations may be either positive (dextro-rotatory—rotate light to the right) or negative (laevorotatory), the direction in which the sugar rotates light may be either the same as, or opposite to, that of the D-/L- (configurational) centre. It is therefore possible to have D-sugars (e.g. fructose) that rotate light to the left and *vice versa*, so the prefixes D- or L- refer *only* to the configuration of the sugar and not to its optical rotation.

Most of the biologically important sugars belong to the D-series, although some L-sugars are also found. The enzymes for metabolism of the sugars are specific for the naturally-occurring forms. Thus glucose oxidase will oxidize D-glucose but not L-glucose.

Cyclic forms

Monosaccharides with five or more carbons usually exist in cyclic (ring) forms. They contain an oxygen bridge between the carbon atom bearing the carbonyl group and another carbon further down the chain. The most common cyclic forms are those with either five or six atoms in the ring. They are referred to as *furanose* or *pyranose* rings respectively, after the names (furan and pyran) of the parent compounds containing such rings.

Chemically, these sugar rings are cyclic hemiacetals. Hemiacetals are formed in reactions between carbonyl compounds (aldehydes or ketones) and alcohols:

$$R\!-\!CHO + HO\!-\!R' \rightleftharpoons R\!-\!\underset{\underset{OH}{|}}{\overset{\overset{H}{|}}{C}}\!-\!O\!-\!R'$$

In sugars, the alcohol group comes from the same molecule as the carbonyl group, so a cyclic compound is formed. In most sugars with five or more carbons, ring formation is favoured because such forms have lower energies than the *aldehydo* or *keto* forms.

In the cyclic forms of sugars there is a further complication to the stereoisomerism of the sugars. This is because the carbon originally bearing the carbonyl group (C-1 for glucose) has now become a chiral carbon and can therefore exist in two different optically-active forms. The two possible forms are known as α- and β-*anomers*. The convention used to distinguish between these is that in α-anomers the hydroxyl group of the new asymmetric centre lies on the same side of the chain as the hydroxyl at the D-/L- determining configurational centre. Conversely, in β-anomers the anomeric hydroxyl group is on the opposite side to the D-/L-hydroxyl. The anomeric forms of D-glucose in both furanose and pyranose rings are shown in figure 1.3A.

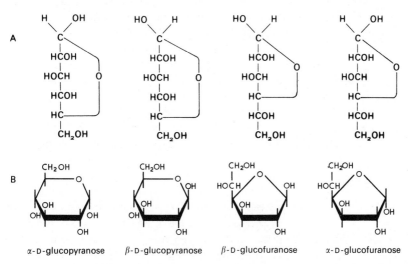

Figure 1.3   Cyclic forms of D-glucose. (A) Projection formulae. (B) Haworth formulae.

One difference between the isomerism due to ring formation and the stereoisomerism at other chiral carbons is that the anomers are much more easily interconverted through the free aldehyde or ketone forms. Such interconversions take place readily in a few minutes or hours, in aqueous solution at room temperature, and give an equilibrium mixture of the different forms. For D-glucose this is a mixture of all five possible forms (aldehyde, α- and β-pyranose, α- and β-furanose), although the two pyranose forms predominate because, for glucose, these are the lowest-energy forms. The equilibrium mixture in aqueous solution contains about 66% of β-D-glucopyranose, 33% of α-D-glucopyranose and only traces of the other three forms.

When glucose is crystallized from aqueous solution, the α-pyranose form is least soluble. Crystalline glucose therefore consists of pure α-D-glucopyranose. Since this has a different optical rotation from the other forms, the process of equilibration when α-D-glucopyranose is dissolved in water can be followed in a polarimeter. The specific rotation of a freshly prepared solution of α-D-glucopyranose is $+111°$ and this falls to $+53°$ over a period of a few hours at room temperature. (β-D-Glucopyranose has a specific rotation of $+19°$, and the equilibrium rotation is closer to that of the β-form because of its higher concentration in the equilibrium mixture.) This equilibration process is known as *mutarotation* and is characteristic of sugars which form rings.

Because of this reaction, cyclic forms of sugars can equilibrate with the free carbonyl form in solution, and show some of the chemical reactions of aldehydes or ketones. One such reaction is that with copper sulphate in alkaline solution to give cuprous oxide. This forms the basis of some tests for sugars. In such reactions, the sugar acts as a reducing agent, and the term *reducing sugar* can be applied to any sugar capable of giving this reaction. Reducing sugars either have a free carbonyl group or exist in ring forms that can readily give a carbonyl group. Some sugars (e.g. the disaccharide sucrose, p. 17) are non-reducing, and this is because they have their potential carbonyl groups substituted in a chemically stable form.

Haworth formulae

Projection formulae for cyclic forms of monosaccharides, such as those of figure 1.3A, are rather distorted because the bond lengths of the C—O—C bonds of the ring are drawn out of proportion to the other bonds in the molecule. To overcome this, the ring forms of sugars are commonly depicted in Haworth formulae of the type shown in figure 1.3B. These

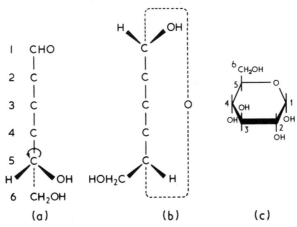

Figure 1.4 Conversion of the projection formula for α-D-glucopyranose to the Haworth formula. In (A) the carbon chain of glucose is shown to emphasize the tetrahedral arrangement at C-5. Free rotation can occur around the C-4 to C-5 bond, and a 120° anticlockwise turn (viewed from above) brings the —OH to behind the molecule (B). This then forms the hemiacetal ring behind the carbon chain to join C-1 to C-5. In the Haworth formula (C) the molecule is turned on its side so that the substituents on the right are now below the plane of the ring.

formulae are three-dimensional representations of the sugar molecules, with the lower edge of the ring nearest the observer and the upper edge further away. To emphasize this, the lower edge is thickened. Substituents are then represented as being either above or below the plane of the ring. Groups that appear to the right in projection formulae are below the plane of the ring in Haworth formulae. Carbons of the ring are not written as such, but are taken to occur at the junction of lines representing bonds. It is also common to omit writing the single hydrogen atoms—these are taken to occur wherever a bond line ends without a specified group.

Carbon 6 of glucose, which was part of the straight chain of carbons in the projection formula, now appears as a substituent above the plane of the ring in the Haworth formula. This transition is illustrated in figure 1.4, where the tetrahedrally arranged substituents around carbon 5 have to be visualized in three dimensions. If difficulty is found in following this, it can be demonstrated with the use of molecular models.

Naturally-occurring monosaccharides

Although there are sixteen sugars in the aldohexose series, only three of these are found commonly in nature. These are D-glucose, D-galactose

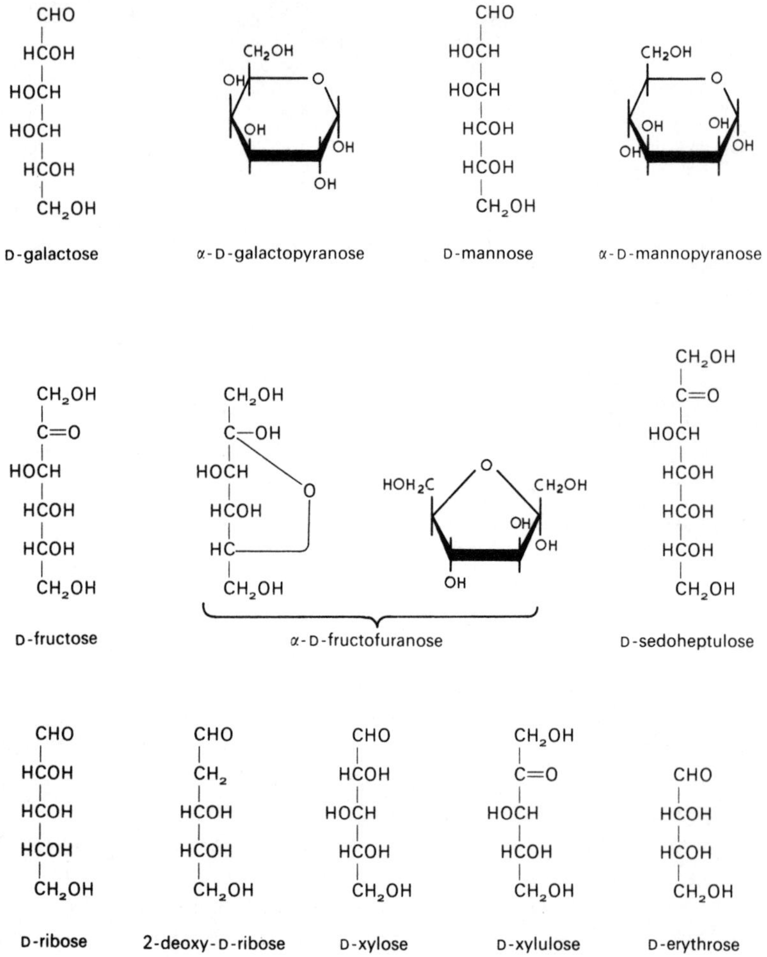

CHO
HCOH
HOCH
HOCH
HCOH
CH$_2$OH

D-galactose

α-D-galactopyranose

CHO
HOCH
HOCH
HCOH
HCOH
CH$_2$OH

D-mannose

α-D-mannopyranose

CH$_2$OH
C=O
HOCH
HCOH
HCOH
CH$_2$OH

D-fructose

α-D-fructofuranose

CH$_2$OH
C=O
HOCH
HCOH
HCOH
HCOH
CH$_2$OH

D-sedoheptulose

CHO
HCOH
HCOH
HCOH
CH$_2$OH

D-ribose

CHO
CH$_2$
HCOH
HCOH
CH$_2$OH

2-deoxy-D-ribose

CHO
HCOH
HOCH
HCOH
CH$_2$OH

D-xylose

CH$_2$OH
C=O
HOCH
HCOH
CH$_2$OH

D-xylulose

CHO
HCOH
HCOH
CH$_2$OH

D-erythrose

Figure 1.5 Some naturally-occurring monosaccharides.

and D-mannose. D-Galactose differs from D-glucose only in its configuration around carbon 4 (figure 1.5) and is therefore a C-4 epimer of
D-glucose. Similarly, D-mannose is a C-2 epimer of D-glucose as it differs
from D-glucose only in the configuration at C-2.

D-Fructose is a ketohexose and, in common with most naturally-
occurring ketoses, the ketone group is at carbon 2. Fructose differs from
glucose in having the carbonyl group at carbon 2 instead of carbon 1, but

the configurations around carbons 3 to 6 are identical in the two sugars. Note that, in the Haworth formula for α-D-fructofuranose, neither carbon 1 nor carbon 6 are part of the ring, and both appear as substituents above the plane of the ring.

Figure 1.5 also shows the structures of some other naturally-occurring sugars which have four, five or seven carbons. D-Erythrose is an aldotetrose; D-ribose and D-xylose are aldopentoses; D-xylulose is a keto-pentose and D-sedoheptulose is a ketoheptose. All of these sugars are important in phosphorylated forms as intermediates in photosynthesis (chapter 4) and in the pentose phosphate pathway (chapter 3).

In *deoxy* sugars, one of the hydroxyl groups of a monosaccharide is replaced by a hydrogen atom as in 2-deoxy D-ribose. D-Ribose and 2-deoxy D-ribose are components of nucleotides and nucleic acids: RNA (ribonucleic acid) contains ribose, and DNA (deoxyribonucleic acid) contains deoxyribose.

Sugar conformation

The angle between bonds in tetrahedral carbon is 109°, whereas the internal angles of a regular hexagon are 120°. Cyclic compounds with rings of six saturated carbons would be under considerable strain if they occurred as flat hexagons, because of distortion of the bond angles of the carbons. Therefore, such compounds relieve the strain by taking up non-planar shapes (or *conformations*), where the bond angles are close to the tetrahedral angle of 109°. Replacement of one of the carbon atoms of such a compound by an oxygen has only a relatively small effect on the ring shape, so the pyranose rings of sugars also take up non-planar conformations.

Figure 1.6 shows some of the possible conformational forms of β-D-glucopyranose. In these, the substituents can either lie in approximately

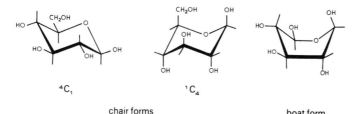

| chair forms | boat form |

Figure 1.6 Conformations of β-D-glucopyranose. The term $^4C_1$ refers to a chair form in which carbon 4 is above, and carbon 1 below, the plane of the molecule.

the same plane as the ring (in the *equatorial* position) or approximately vertically above or below the ring (in the *axial* position). When several large substituents are present in axial positions, they tend to repel each other but, if the same groups are present in equatorial positions, they are further separated, so that there is less interaction between them. This means that the preferred conformation is usually that in which the majority of the large substituents are in equatorial positions. In the two chair forms of β-D-glucopyranose shown in figure 1.6, one conformation ($^4C_1$) has all the large substituent groups in equatorial positions whereas, in the other conformation ($^1C_4$), they are all in axial positions. From the generalization made above, it is apparent that the $^4C_1$ form is the

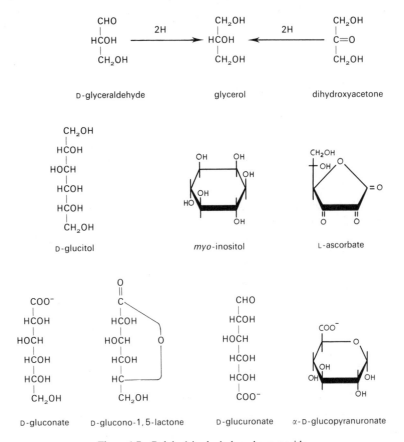

Figure 1.7 Polyhydric alcohols and sugar acids.

preferred conformation and the one in which most molecules will be present most of the time.

It should be noted that changes in conformation do not involve the breaking of any covalent bonds, but only rotation around bonds. Changes in conformation can occur rapidly in solution, so that a sugar will be present as a mixture of different conformational forms with the equilibrium favouring the lowest-energy forms. However, some of the other forms may be important for biochemical reactions of the sugars, and there is evidence that the conformation of carbohydrate substrates is altered during the formation of certain enzyme-substrate complexes. Such a conformation change occurs during polysaccharide hydrolysis by lysozyme.

The conformation of sugars is of importance in its effect on the equilibrium position of chemical and biochemical interconversion of sugars. In the mutarotation of glucose (p. 6), the equilibrium somewhat favours the β-pyranose form, because it can take up a $^4C_1$ conformation in which all substituents are equatorial whereas, in the α-pyranose form, the hydroxyl group at C-1 is axial. Similarly, in the biological interconversion of derivatives of D-glucose and D-galactose (p. 51), the equilibrium mixture contains rather more of the glucose derivative with an equatorial hydroxyl group than of the galactose derivative which has an axial group at C-4.

Furanose rings are also found in different conformational forms but, because such rings are more nearly flat than pyranose rings, the energy differences between the different forms are not as great. Consequently, in solution, the furanose sugars are often an equilibrium mixture of rather similar proportions of several conformational forms.

Sugar alcohols

Sugar alcohols (polyhydric alcohols, polyols) may be formed by reduction of the carbonyl group of a sugar to a hydroxyl group. Thus glycerol can be formed by reduction of glyceraldehyde or by reduction of the keto-triose dihydroxyacetone (figure 1.7). D-Glucitol (also known as sorbitol) is similarly formed from D-glucose.

Keto sugars can give more than one sugar alcohol. Thus chemical reduction of D-fructose introduces a new chiral centre at C-2 and results in a mixture of D-glucitol and D-mannitol.

Glycerol is important as a component of lipids, where it may be esterified directly to fatty acids as in the triglycerides, or it may be linked through a phosphate group to other components as in the phospholipids. Glycerol and glucitol are also found in large quantities in the over-wintering stages of some insects. Here they act as antifreeze agents by depressing the freezing-point of body fluids and by enhancing their supercooling properties.

The sugar alcohols derived from reducing sugars can occur only in the straight-chain form, because the carbonyl group required to form the cyclic hemiacetal rings is absent. There is, however, a related group of cyclic compounds (known as the cyclitols) which have a ring consisting of only carbon atoms, each of which bears a hydroxyl group. The most important of these compounds is *myo*-inositol (figure 1.7) which is a component of phospholipids.

Sugar acids

Sugar acids are formed when one or other of the terminal carbons of a sugar is oxidized to a carboxylic acid group. This gives two series of sugar acids:

(1) In the *aldonic* acids, the carboxylic acid group is at carbon 1, and such compounds are formed by oxidizing the aldehyde group of an aldo-sugar. Thus D-gluconic acid is formed by oxidation of D-glucose at carbon 1. In the aldonic acids, the main functional group is a carboxylic acid group instead of an aldehyde. Aldonic acids can form rings, but these are chemically different from the hemiacetal rings of the reducing sugars. Such rings are cyclic esters ("lactones") formed between the carboxylic acid group and one of the hydroxyl groups in the same molecule to give either a five- or a six-membered ring. The six-membered ring form of D-gluconic acid is D-glucono-1,5-lactone and is shown in figure 1.7.

(2) The *uronic* acids are monosaccharide derivatives in which a carboxylic acid group is present at the highest-numbered carbon of the sugar. This leaves the aldehyde group unchanged at C-1, so the uronic acids can still form cyclic hemiacetal rings through this group. They are also able to form glycosidic links with other sugars, and this property makes them important as components of polysaccharides where they are able to confer acidic character to the molecules (chapter 8). Figure 1.7 shows D-glucuronic acid, which is the uronic acid corresponding to D-glucose. At physiological pH, such acids are present in the ionized form. They are shown in this form in figure 1.7 and are referred to as ions (e.g. D-glucuronate) rather than as acids.

The *aldaric* acids are sugar derivatives with carboxylic acid groups at both ends of the carbon chain. These compounds are not of biological importance. Another oxidation product of monosaccharides is L-ascorbate (also known as vitamin C, p. 59).

Amino sugars

Amino sugars are formed by replacement of one of the hydroxyl groups of a sugar by an amino group. In many of the amino sugars, it is the hydroxyl group attached to carbon 2 which is replaced. Figure 1.8 shows the structure of D-glucosamine (2-amino 2-deoxy D-glucose) which is the amino sugar derived from D-glucose.

The main function of amino sugars in biology is as components of polysaccharides, and here they are often present as their *N*-acetyl derivatives. Figure 1.8 shows the structure of *N*-acetyl D-glucosamine and of two more complex amino sugars—neuraminate and muramate.

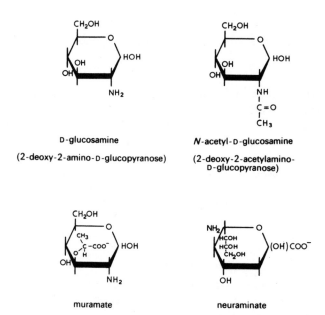

Figure 1.8 Amino sugars. Note that, when the anomeric position of a sugar is not substituted, the configuration at this position is not specified, because the molecules can exist as a mixture of α- and β-forms.

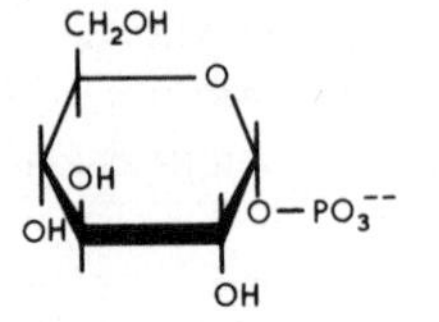

glucose 1-phosphate

(α-D-glucopyranosyl phosphate)

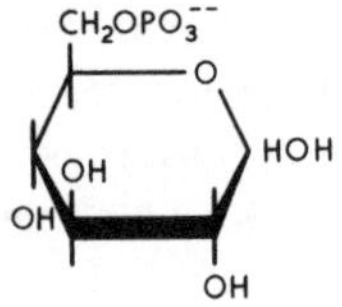

glucose 6-phosphate

(6-phospho-D-glucopyranose)

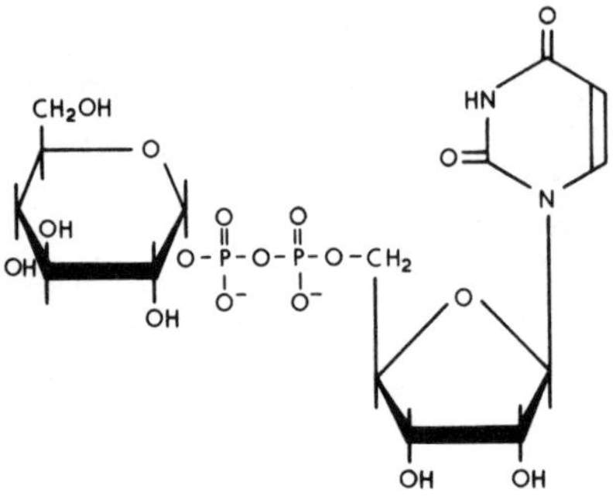

uridine diphosphate glucose (UDP-Glc)

Figure 1.9   Sugar phosphates and nucleoside diphosphate sugars.

Sugar phosphates

The first step in the metabolism of sugars is nearly always formation of a sugar phosphate derivative. Such compounds are intermediates in glycolysis and most other metabolic pathways of carbohydrate metabolism. In sugar phosphates, an orthophosphate group may be esterified either to the primary hydroxyl group (as in glucose 6-phosphate) or to the anomeric hydroxyl group (as in glucose 1-phosphate) (figure 1.9).

Note that, in glucose 1-phosphate, the phosphate group may be either in the α- or β-position, and that the two forms are not interconverted in solution (p. 6). This is because interconversion of anomeric forms of free sugars takes place through the free carbonyl forms and requires the presence of an unsubstituted anomeric hydroxyl group. Substitution of this hydroxyl group by phosphate, or any other group, prevents ring opening and equilibration of anomers. Sugars substituted at the anomeric carbon no longer have the reducing properties of free sugars, such as the ability to reduce cupric salts in alkaline solution.

Related to the sugar phosphates is another group of sugar derivatives known as the nucleoside diphosphate sugars. In these compounds, the monosaccharide is linked through the anomeric position to a nucleoside diphosphate, as shown for uridine diphosphate glucose (UDP-Glc) in figure 1.9. These derivatives are important as coenzymes in the biological interconversion of sugars (chapter 3) and in the synthesis of glycosides (chapter 6).

Glycosides

Glycosides are formed when the anomeric hydroxyl of a sugar reacts with a hydroxyl group of a second molecule with the elimination of water. This reaction results in a glycosidic linkage between the two molecules.

Figure 1.10 shows an example of glycoside formation. When glucose is heated in methanol in the presence of acid catalyst, a mixture of methyl glucosides is formed. The major products of this reaction are the α- and β-pyranosides, but smaller amounts of the furanosides are also formed.

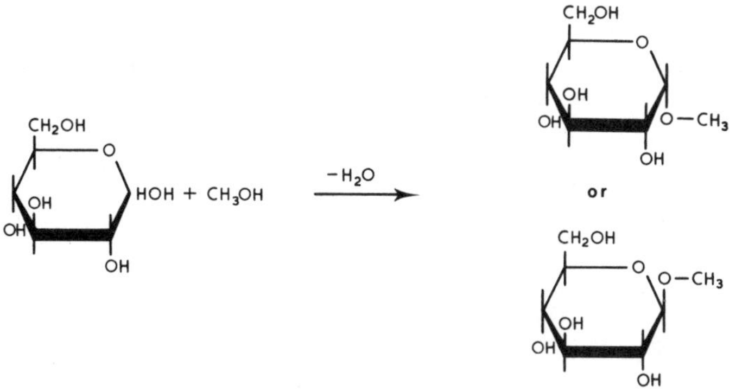

Figure 1.10   Reaction of glucose with methanol in the presence of a catalyst gives a mixture of methyl α-D-glucopyranoside and methyl β-D-glucopyranoside.

Once the anomeric hydroxyl group has been substituted, the anomeric form and ring size of the derivative is fixed. Thus crystalline methyl α-D-glucopyranoside when dissolved in water does not show mutarotation but remains in the α-pyranose form.

Glycoside formation is a special case of acetal formation. Acetals are formed from carbonyl compounds and alcohols in a two-stage reaction:

$$\text{(1)} \qquad R\text{—}CHO + HO\text{—}R' \rightleftharpoons R\text{—}\underset{\underset{OH}{|}}{\overset{\overset{H}{|}}{C}}\text{—}O\text{—}R' \quad \text{(hemiacetal)}$$

$$(2) \qquad R{-}\overset{\overset{\displaystyle H}{|}}{\underset{\underset{\displaystyle OH}{|}}{C}}{-}O{-}R + HO{-}R'' \rightleftharpoons R{-}\overset{\overset{\displaystyle H}{|}}{\underset{\underset{\displaystyle O{-}R''}{|}}{C}}{-}O{-}R' + H_2O \quad \text{(acetal)}$$

In sugars, the first step corresponds to ring formation, and the second step to glycoside formation.

Disaccharides

Disaccharides are glycosides containing two monosaccharide residues. The anomeric carbon of one of the monosaccharides is glycosidically linked to one of the carbons of the other monosaccharide. Since there are usually several hydroxyl groups on the second monosaccharide, there are several ways of joining two monosaccharides together, and therefore a number of different disaccharides can be produced. Note that the anomeric carbon of at least one of the sugars must be involved in the glycosidic link.

Some examples of disaccharides are given in figure 1.11. In maltose, the anomeric carbon of one glucose residue (on the left) is joined through an oxygen to carbon 4 of the other glucose residue. The linkage is α with respect to carbon 1 of the first sugar, so it is described as an $\alpha(1 \rightarrow 4)$

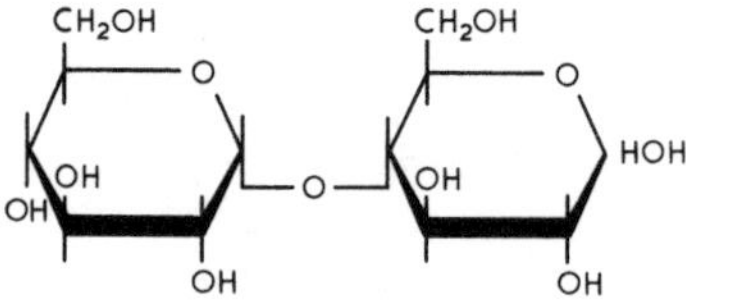

(a) maltose

(O-α-D-glucopyranosyl-(1→4)-D-glucopyranose)

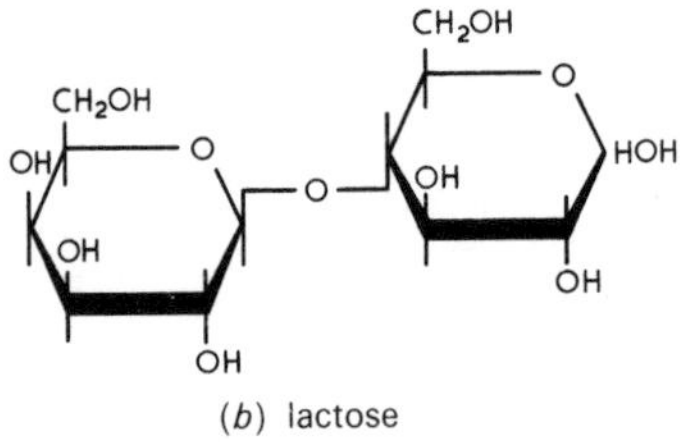

(b) lactose

(O-β-D-galactopyranosyl-(1→4)-D-glucopyranose)

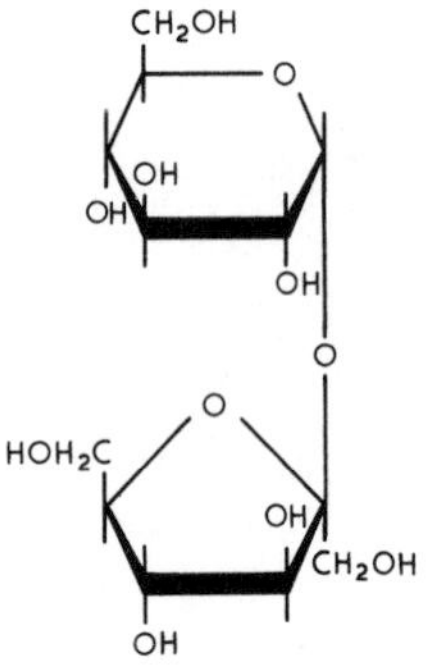

(c) sucrose

(O-β-D-fructofuranosyl-α-D-glucopyranoside)

Figure 1.11   Disaccharides.

linkage. The full name for maltose is O-α-D-glucopyranosyl-(1 → 4)-D-glucopyranose. The first part of the name applies to the left-hand sugar of the figure, and the ending -osyl shows that this sugar contributes the anomeric carbon to the linkage. The second part of the name refers to the right-hand sugar, and the ending -ose implies that the anomeric hydroxyl of this sugar is unsubstituted.

Maltose is a reducing sugar by virtue of its unsubstituted carbon 1 and, in solution, will equilibrate to a mixture of α- and β-pyranose forms at the right-hand glucose unit (but not at the left-hand glucose). An important feature of the free anomeric hydroxyl of maltose is that this is capable of forming a glycosidic link with a further glucose, and it is in this way that extended chains of sugars can be joined together to form polysaccharides.

In lactose (figure 1.11b), two different monosaccharides are linked together. The galactose residue (on the left in the figure) is joined through its anomeric carbon at C-1 through a β-linkage to C-4 of a glucose residue. Lactose is also a reducing disaccharide because the anomeric group of the glucose residue is not substituted.

Sucrose (figure 1.11c) is a disaccharide in which glucose and fructose are joined together through their anomeric carbons. Since the reducing groups of both monosaccharides are involved in the glycosidic link, both are "fixed" in their respective forms—α-pyranose for glucose and β-furanose for fructose—and sucrose is a non-reducing sugar.

Polysaccharides

Polysaccharides contain many monosaccharide residues joined together through glycosidic links. Some, like amylose (p. 118), are relatively simple in structure and have identical monosaccharide residues joined into long chains by identical types of glycosidic links. Others, like glycogen (p. 108), have branched structures in which two types of glycosidic link occur. More complex polysaccharides contain several different types of monosaccharide glycosidically linked in different ways, and may also be covalently joined to proteins or lipids. Examples of these different types of polysaccharide will be considered in greater detail in chapters 8 and 9.

Nomenclature and abbreviations

Table 1.1 summarizes some of the more common terms used in carbohydrate nomenclature, and table 1.2 gives some abbreviations in common usage.

Table 1.1 Common terms used in carbohydrate chemistry

Term	Meaning
Glycoside	Compound in which H of hemiacetyl —OH is replaced by aryl or alkyl residue. Named by substituting -ide in place of -e as suffix to name of monosaccharide, e.g. galactoside.
Glycosyl	General term for a glycosidically-linked group, e.g. galactosyl, mannosyl.
Aglycone	Group in a glycoside to which the glycosyl group is linked.
Anomeric carbon, glycosidic carbon	Carbon atom bearing a carbonyl group or potential carbonyl group through which cyclic forms and glycosides can be formed.
Configurational centre, reference carbon	Highest numbered asymmetric centre, at which the configuration determines the D/L classification.
Glucan, arabinan, etc.	Polysaccharide of glucose, arabinose, etc.

Table 1.2 Common abbreviations used in carbohydrate chemistry

Common sugars: D-glucose	Glc	
D-mannose	Man	
D-galactose	Gal	
D-fructose	Fru	
D-ribose	Rib	
D-arabinose	Ara	
D-xylose	Xyl	
L-fucose	Fuc	(6-deoxy-L-galactose)
N-acetyl neuraminate	AcNeu	

Cyclic forms: Use suffix *p* for pyranose or *f* for furanose, e.g. Glc*p*.
Uronic acids: Use suffix A, e.g. GalA (or Gal*p*A).
Amino sugars: Use suffix N, e.g. ManN (or Man*p*N).
N-Acetyl amino sugars: Use suffix NAc, e.g. GlcNAc.
Glycosides: Glycosyl group is written on left, then anomeric configuration, then (in parentheses) the positions joining the two groups are indicated with an arrow pointing from the glycosyl group, then the aglycone, e.g. maltose: Glc*p*α(1 → 4)Glc.
Sugar phosphates: Use *P* for orthophosphate group —PO_3^{--}, e.g. Glc 6-*P*.
Inorganic orthophosphate: Use Pi.
Inorganic pyrophosphate: Use PPi.
Deoxy sugars: Use prefix d, e.g. dRib.

Where there is no ambiguity, the prefixes D- and L- may be omitted from names of carbohydrates used in biological descriptions, so that "glucose" is commonly used for D-glucose.

In phosphorylated derivatives, the term *bisphosphate* (as in fructose 1,6-bisphosphate) is used to describe a derivative in which two orthophosphate groups are attached at separate positions to the sugar, whereas the term *diphosphate* is reserved for compounds containing a pyrophosphate group as in adenosine diphosphate.

CHAPTER TWO

GLYCOLYSIS

Glycolysis is the most widely-occurring pathway for the breakdown of carbohydrate, and is found in most animals and plants and in many bacteria. It was one of the first major metabolic pathways to be elucidated, and is named the "Embden-Meyerhof-Parnas" pathway after investigators who made major contributions to its discovery in the 1930s. The term *glycolysis* means "splitting of sugar" and the process results in cleavage of the hexose molecule into two three-carbon fragments.

The most important function of glycolysis is in energy metabolism. The conversion of carbohydrates to pyruvate in glycolysis is an exergonic process because the substrate has a higher energy of combustion than the products. This is partly due to a regrouping of hydrogen and oxygen atoms from hydroxyl and carbonyl groups to give the lower-energy carboxylate group. To make use of the available energy, it is necessary to collect it in a form in which it can be made use of by the cell. All cells use ATP for this purpose, and couple reactions such as glycolysis to the synthesis of ATP from ADP plus inorganic orthophosphate. The subsequent conversion of ATP to ADP is a thermodynamically favourable reaction which can be used to carry out work by coupling it to what otherwise would be thermodynamically unfavourable reactions. Thus ATP is hydrolysed during mechanical work (as in muscle contraction) and is used for chemical work required for synthetic reactions and for transport of solutes across the cell membrane. ATP is also used in such varied reactions as light emission in fireflies and for electricity generation in electric eels. ATP forms a common currency linking the energy-requiring reactions to reactions in which the "fuels" such as carbohydrates are degraded.

Another function of glycolysis in many cells is the conversion of carbohydrates to pyruvate, which can then provide substrate for the oxidative reactions of the tricarboxylic acid cycle. Glycolysis and the tricarboxylic acid cycle can function as a unit for the complete oxidation of carbohydrate to carbon dioxide and water, both pathways contributing to energy metabolism by being coupled to ATP synthesis. However, in some cells, glycolysis can operate independently of the tricarboxylic acid cycle, and this is particularly important under conditions where oxygen is not available for pyruvate oxidation (p. 31).

A third function for glycolysis is in the synthesis of substrates for synthetic reactions such as formation of lipids and of some amino acids; for example, the glycerol component of triglycerides is synthesized by reduction of the triose phosphate intermediates of glycolysis.

Substrates for glycolysis

Many carbohydrates can be used by different organisms as substrates for glycolysis, but the most common are glucose and the polysaccharides glycogen and starch. Glucose is an exogenous substrate, that is, it is present in the environment of the cell, whether it be the growth medium of a microorganism or the blood of a vertebrate animal. The first step in its metabolism is transport across the plasma membrane into the cell. This process is considered further in chapter 5. Glycogen and starch are storage polysaccharides whose function is to act as endogenous substrate within the cells (chapter 7), and they may be metabolized without intervention of a transport step. For short periods, the cell can operate independently of an external carbohydrate supply by using its stored polysaccharide.

Other substrates for glycolysis include hexoses such as fructose, galactose and mannose. Mechanisms for the conversion of different sugars into the sugar phosphate intermediates of glycolysis will be considered further in chapter 3. The disaccharide sucrose is used for transporting carbohydrates to different tissues in plants, and so can be a glycolytic substrate for plant cells, and a similar role is played by another disaccharide, trehalose in insects (chapter 6). Microorganisms are able to use a variety of different sugars supplied in the growth medium, and adapt to using new sugars by synthesizing specific enzymes capable of metabolizing them.

The reactions of glycolysis

An outline of the sequence of reactions which constitute the pathway of glycolysis is shown in figure 2.1. The operation of the pathway as a whole

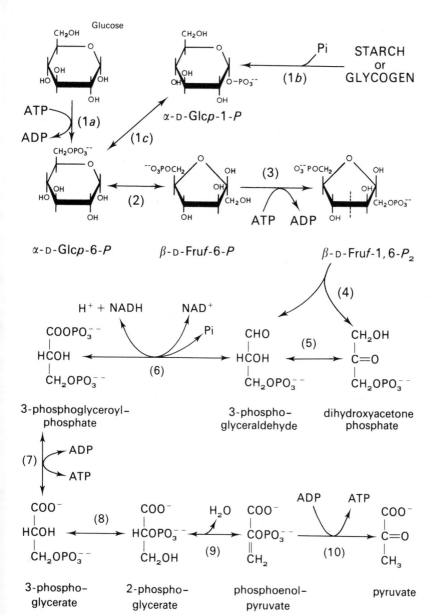

Figure 2.1 The reactions of glycolysis. The enzymes are: (1a) hexokinase; (1b) phosphorylase; (1c) phosphoglucomutase; (2) phosphoglucose isomerase; (3) 6-phosphofructokinase; (4) aldolase; (5) triosephosphate isomerase; (6) glyceraldehydephosphate dehydrogenase; (7) phosphoglycerate kinase; (8) phosphoglycerate mutase; (9) enolase; (10) pyruvate kinase.

will be discussed later in the chapter, but the individual reactions and the enzymes that catalyse them are first considered in more detail.

Hexokinase

The first step in the metabolism of sugars is usually their phosphorylation, and hexokinase catalyses a typical reaction for the conversion of sugars to their phosphate derivatives. Both α- and β-anomers of D-glucopyranose are phosphorylated specifically at the C-6 hydroxyl group by transfer of the terminal phosphate group of ATP onto the sugar substrate. (ATP is the phosphate group donor in all reactions catalysed by "kinases".) The equilibrium of this reaction is greatly in favour of sugar phosphate formation, especially at the high ATP/ADP ratio found in most cells, so the reaction is irreversible under physiological conditions. Magnesium ions are required for the reaction, because the true substrate is the magnesium complex of ATP ($MgATP^{--}$).

Four different isoenzymes of hexokinase (types I–IV) are found in mammals, and different tissues contain their own characteristic iso-enzyme(s). Thus skeletal muscle contains type II, whereas liver contains type IV in highest activity. Types I to III are rather similar to each other in having a low K_m for glucose of 10^{-6} to 10^{-4} M and in showing inhibition by glucose 6-phosphate, the product of the reaction. This inhibition is believed to be important in the regulation of glycolysis (p. 38). The fourth hexokinase isoenzyme (type IV, "glucokinase") has a high K_m for glucose of about 10^{-2} M and is not inhibited by glucose 6-phosphate. This enzyme is involved in the metabolism of blood glucose when this becomes elevated after intake of a carbohydrate-containing meal. The hexokinases of other organisms usually resemble the types I to III hexokinases of mammals in showing a low K_m for glucose and inhibition by glucose 6-phosphate. In some mammalian tissues (liver and brain), hexokinase is partly associated with the mitochondria, and the intracellular distribution may be important in the regulation of glucose phosphorylation.

Some bacteria use an additional mechanism to phosphorylate glucose. Here transport of the sugar into the cell is coupled to its phosphorylation in a reaction which uses phosphoenolpyruvate as phosphate donor (p. 92).

Phosphoglucomutase

The phosphoglucomutase reaction is an essential step linking glycogen metabolism with glycolysis. Thus the product of phosphorylase action on glycogen is glucose 1-phosphate (p. 112) which must first be converted to glucose 6-phosphate by phosphoglucomutase before it can be metabolized by subsequent reactions of glycolysis.

The enzyme from rabbit muscle has a serine residue which can be esterified by a phosphate group to give phospho-enzyme. In this form the enzyme is capable of converting either glucose 1-phosphate or glucose 6-phosphate to the enzyme-bound intermediate, glucose 1,6-bisphosphate. This can dissociate from the enzyme to give free glucose 1,6-bisphosphate and dephospho-enzyme, but free glucose 1,6-bisphosphate is not a mandatory intermediate in the conversion of glucose 1-phosphate to glucose 6-phosphate. The reaction can be summarized as follows:

$$\text{Enz-}P + \text{Glc-1-}P \rightleftharpoons \text{Enz-Glc-1,6-}P_2 \rightleftharpoons \text{Enz-}P + \text{Glc-6-}P$$
$$\updownarrow$$
$$\text{Enz} + \text{Glc-1,6-}P_2$$

During the interconversion, the substrate receives a new phosphate group from the phosphoenzyme and, in turn, leaves its own phosphate group behind on the enzyme.

Phosphoglucomutase is specific for α-D-glucopyranosyl phosphate, which is the isomer of glucose 1-phosphate produced during the phosphorylase reaction. At equilibrium, the reaction mixture contains 95% glucose 6-phosphate and 5% glucose 1-phosphate, and in many cells the enzyme is sufficiently active to maintain a ratio of glucose phosphate concentrations similar to these equilibrium proportions.

Glucosephosphate isomerase

Glucosephosphate isomerase catalyses the reversible interconversion of the 6-phosphates of glucose and fructose:

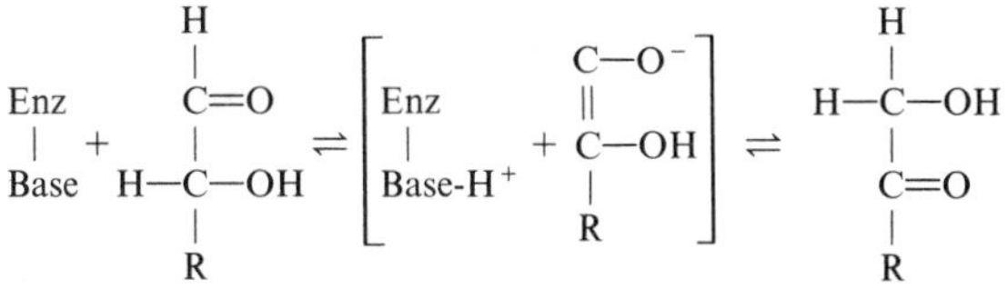

The reaction is base-catalysed by a basic imidazole (histidine) residue in the enzyme, and an enediol is formed as an enzyme-bound intermediate. This seems to be a general mechanism for ketone-aldehyde interconversions (p. 48).

The enzyme can act on either the α- or β-anomers of glucopyranose

6-phosphate, and also has the ability to catalyse the interconversion of different forms of both substrates with the open-chain forms by an "anomerase" (mutarotase) activity. This is important to the action of the enzyme, because the interconversion takes place through the acyclic forms. Like phosphoglucomutase, the enzyme is usually present in cells in fairly high activity, so that the ratio of glucose 6-phosphate to fructose 6-phosphate in tissues tends to be similar to the equilibrium ratio of approximately 2:1.

6-Phosphofructokinase

Phosphofructokinase catalyses the ATP-dependent phosphorylation of the C-1 hydroxyl of fructose 6-phosphate to give fructose 1,6-bisphosphate. The enzyme is specific for the β-furanose form of the substrate and gives the corresponding form of the product. The equilibrium of the reaction is strongly in favour of fructose 1,6-bisphosphate formation, and in most cells the reaction does not approach equilibrium because the activity of the enzyme is low relative to most other enzymes of glycolysis. The rate of this reaction therefore often limits the rate of flow of substrates through glycolysis. For this reason, the phosphofructokinase reaction is a control point for glycolysis, and the enzyme is subject to regulation through a number of different effectors (p. 38).

Aldolase

In the aldolase reaction, fructose 1,6-bisphosphate is split to give the two triose phosphates, dihydroxyacetone phosphate (from C-1 to C-3 of fructose) and D-glyceraldehyde 3-phosphate (from C-4 to C-6 of fructose). The equilibrium of this reaction is rather unusual in that it depends upon the actual concentrations of substrate and products—the lower the substrate concentrations, the higher the relative proportions of triose phosphates. This is because the reaction has one substrate and two products, so the equilibrium is represented by:

$$K = \frac{[\text{DHAP}] \times [\text{Gly-3-}P]}{[\text{Fru-1,6-}P_2]} \quad (= \text{approx. } 10^{-4}\,\text{M})$$

Since the triose phosphates are equilibrated through the triose phosphate isomerase reaction, the numerator of the equilibrium equation is equivalent to the square of the total triose phosphate concentration. Thus, if the equilibrium is to be maintained, any change in the fructose 1,6-bisphosphate concentration must be matched by a change in triose phosphate concentration equal to the square root of the change in fructose bisphosphate; for example, a 100-fold decrease in fructose bisphosphate would be balanced by a 10-fold decrease in triose phosphate. At the concentrations of reactants normally found in cells, the aldolase reaction is close to equilibrium. Aldolase can act either on the β-furanose form of the substrate (the form produced by the preceding phosphofructokinase reaction) or on the acyclic ketone form.

Triose phosphate isomerase

Further metabolism of the triose phosphates by glycolysis occurs via D-glyceraldehyde 3-phosphate, so, for complete metabolism of substrate, the dihydroxyacetone phosphate produced at the aldolase step must be converted to glyceraldehyde phosphate. The triose phosphate isomerase reaction resembles that of glucosephosphate isomerase in that aldose and ketose phosphates are interconverted (p. 48).

Glyceraldehyde 3-phosphate dehydrogenase

In this reaction, the oxidation of D-glyceraldehyde 3-phosphate takes place at C-1, and phosphate is also incorporated into the molecule at the same position. The product, 3-phospho-D-glyceroylphosphate, is a derivative of D-glyceric acid containing one phosphate group esterified at C-3, and another phosphate group as a mixed anhydride between the carboxylate group at C-1 and orthophosphate.

A cysteine residue of the enzyme is involved in binding the substrate as a thiohemiacetal intermediate (figure 2.2). The reaction proceeds by substrate oxidation with NAD^+ (also bound to the enzyme) to give the thioester of 3-phosphoglycerate. The enzyme-bound NADH produced is then displaced by NAD^+, and the phosphoglycerate is transferred from thioester onto inorganic phosphate.

The glyceraldehyde phosphate dehydrogenase reaction is sensitive to inhibition by iodoacetate because of a selective reaction of this reagent with the sulphydryl group of the reactive cysteine group of the enzyme. Iodoacetate and similar reagents have been used experimentally to inhibit glycolysis, although the inhibition is not quite selective enough to be completely specific. Arsenate also interferes with the reaction by replacing phosphate as the acceptor of the oxidized substrate. Unlike the corresponding phosphate derivative, the 3-phosphoglyceroyl arsenate produced is rapidly and non-enzymically hydrolysed to 3-phosphoglycerate, so the reaction is non-productive in terms of eventual ATP synthesis.

The equilibrium of the glyceraldehyde phosphate dehydrogenase reaction is such that at equal concentrations of NAD^+ and NADH the proportion of glyceraldehyde phosphate greatly exceeds that of 3-phosphoglyceroyl phosphate. However, the mass action effect of the high NAD^+/NADH ratio in the cytosol (about 1000/1 in liver) alters the equilibrium proportions of the phosphates such that 3-phosphoglyceroyl phosphate formation is more favoured.

In some cells glyceraldehyde phosphate dehydrogenase comprises between 10 and 20% of the total soluble protein.

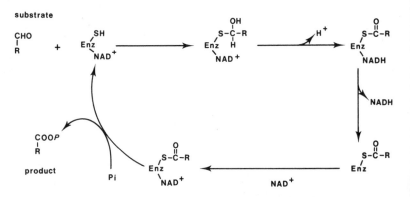

Figure 2.2   Intermediates of the glyceraldehydephosphate dehydrogenase reaction.

$$R = H\overset{|}{C}OH$$
$$CH_2OP$$

Phosphoglycerate kinase

In this reaction, there is a direct transfer of the phosphate group from the substrate onto ADP to give ATP. This general type of reaction for the phosphorylation of ADP is known as "substrate level phosphorylation" to distinguish it from oxidative phosphorylation which occurs in association with electron transport in mitochondria. The reaction catalysed by phosphoglycerate kinase is close to equilibrium under most physiological conditions.

Phosphoglyceromutase

The isomerization of 3-phosphoglycerate and 2-phosphoglycerate has some similarity to the isomerization of glucose phosphates by the phosphoglucomutase reaction. 2,3-Bisphosphoglycerate is required as cofactor, and the mechanism can be represented as:

$$
\begin{array}{cccc}
\text{COO}^- & \text{COO}^- & \text{COO}^- & \text{COO}^- \\
| & | & | & | \\
\text{HCOH} + \text{HCO}P & \rightleftharpoons \text{HCO}P & + \text{HCO}P \\
| & | & | & | \\
\text{CH}_2 O P & \text{CH}_2 O P & \text{CH}_2\text{OH} & \text{CH}_2 O P
\end{array}
$$

Each molecule of substrate passes through the intermediate 2,3-bisphosphoglycerate stage during the interconversion.

Enolase

Enolase catalyses the removal of water from 2-phosphoglycerate to give phosphoenolpyruvate. Although there is no overall oxidation of substrate in this reaction, it can be considered that C-3 has been reduced (by removal of —OH) at the expense of oxidation at C-2 (by removal of H), so that the group bearing the phosphate is converted to a more oxidized form.

This enzyme requires a divalent cation such as Mg^{++} for its activity. The inhibitory effect of fluoride on glycolysis is due to a reaction between fluoride, magnesium ions and orthophosphate to give a magnesium fluorophosphate complex, thereby removing magnesium ions from the solution.

Pyruvate kinase

The pyruvate kinase reaction is the second step of glycolysis at which ATP is generated, and the other product (pyruvate) is the first non-phosphorylated intermediate to arise. In most cells, the reactants are far removed from the equilibrium position, and the reaction is one of the control points of glycolysis (p. 38).

Energy metabolism

At the beginning of this chapter it was shown that an important function of glycolysis is to synthesize ATP from ADP. The relationship between carbohydrate breakdown and ATP synthesis can now be examined.

The reactions of glycolysis in which ATP is involved as substrate or product are those catalysed by hexokinase, phosphofructokinase, phosphoglycerate kinase and pyruvate kinase. The first two reactions each use one ATP for every molecule of glucose metabolized, whereas the other reactions each generate two ATP molecules for every glucose used. (Note that at reactions beyond aldolase there are two molecules of triose phosphate for each glucose used, so the later reactions have twice as many substrate molecules as the earlier reactions of glycolysis.) There is, therefore, a net synthesis of two molecules of ATP for each glucose metabolized. When glycogen is the substrate, there is a net synthesis of three ATP molecules per hexose. This difference is due to the different initial reactions by which the substrates enter metabolism—glucose is phosphorylated at the expense of ATP in the hexokinase reaction, whereas the phosphorolysis of glycogen requires only inorganic phosphate.

The energy metabolism of the cell depends critically upon the interaction of ATP with other phosphorylated intermediates: some intermediates are used to donate their phosphate group to ADP, whereas others accept phosphate from ATP. The type of reaction capable of taking place under physiological conditions depends partly on the equilibrium constants for the hydrolysis of the phosphorylated compounds. In a transfer reaction between two phosphates, it will be the one whose equilibrium constant for hydrolysis is most strongly in favour of hydrolysis which will donate its phosphate group to the other compound. In other words, the more exergonic is the hydrolysis of a phosphate, the greater is the potential for transferring the phosphate to an acceptor. A knowledge of the equilibrium constants of the hydrolysis of such phosphates is thus useful in predicting the equilibrium of transfer reactions, in particular between ATP and other compounds. The amount of free energy released when ATP is hydrolysed to ADP plus orthophosphate is about 50 kJ per mole, where the concentrations of reactants are approximately the same as those found in an average cell. The hydrolysis of glucose 6-phosphate, however, is only about half as exergonic as for ATP. From this it can be deduced that in the transfer of phosphate from ATP to glucose in the hexokinase reaction, the equilibrium favours glucose 6-phosphate formation at the expense of ATP.

These differences in the free energies of hydrolysis of different phosphate derivatives are due to the different chemical nature of the compounds. Simple phosphate esters such as glucose 6-phosphate, fructose 6-phosphate and 3-phosphoglycerate have relatively low standard free energies of hydrolysis of around 15–25 kJ/mole. However, ATP is an acid anhydride, and its hydrolysis is favoured by additional factors which do not contribute to the hydrolysis of phosphate esters. One factor is that the negative charges on the three phosphate groups of ATP tend to repel each other, so that the substrate is less stable than the hydrolysis products in which the charged groups are separated. Another factor is that the products are able to take up a greater number of resonance forms than the substrate. These factors which favour ATP hydrolysis also affect the equilibria of other reactions in which ATP is converted to ADP, and help to explain why the equilibrium of the hexokinase reaction lies in favour of glucose 6-phosphate formation.

Many of the intermediates of glycolysis are simple phosphate esters and have correspondingly relatively low free energies of hydrolysis. Two of the intermediates, however, have a far higher standard free energy of hydrolysis than the others. These are 3-phosphoglyceroyl phosphate and phosphoenolpyruvate, and it is these compounds that are linked to the phosphorylation of ADP to give ATP.

3-Phosphoglyceroyl phosphate has two phosphate groups, but it is the one in the C-1 position which is important in ATP synthesis, because it is a mixed anhydride between a carboxylic acid and phosphoric acid. The free energy of hydrolysis of this anhydride is rather higher than that of ATP, and it can be used for ADP phosphorylation as in the phosphoglycerate kinase reaction.

The second compound, phosphoenolpyruvate, is a phosphate ester but has a high free energy of hydrolysis because the initial reaction product, *enol*-pyruvate, isomerizes almost completely to the very much more favoured *keto* form. This isomerization involves a large free-energy change, so that the overall standard free energy of hydrolysis of phosphoenolpyruvate is as much as 65 kJ/mole (more than that of ATP). The equilibrium of the pyruvate kinase reaction is considerably in favour of pyruvate and ATP formation, and is a physiologically irreversible reaction.

$$
\begin{array}{ccc}
\text{COO}^- & \text{COO}^- & \text{COO}^- \\
| & | & | \\
\text{CO}P + \text{ADP} \rightleftharpoons \text{ATP} + \text{COH} \rightarrow \text{C}=\text{O} \\
|| & || & | \\
\text{CH}_2 & \text{CH}_2 & \text{CH}_3 \\
\end{array}
$$

phosphoenolpyruvate   enol   keto

pyruvate

These reactions which favour ATP synthesis help to maintain the high concentration of ATP in the cell relative to ADP, so that in many cells nearly 90% of all the adenine nucleotides are present as ATP.

Oxidation-reduction reactions

The oxidation of every molecule of triose phosphate at the glyceraldehyde phosphate dehydrogenase reaction is coupled to the reduction of a molecule of NAD^+ to NADH. Since there is only a small amount of NAD^+ in the cell, the NADH must be reoxidized immediately if glycolysis is to continue. (The total amount of NAD^+ in contracting muscle is only sufficient to allow glycolysis to continue for about one second if no reoxidation were to occur.) It follows that all cells which are capable of glycolysis must also have an efficient mechanism for reoxidation of NADH. Several different reactions are used for this, and they can be divided into two main groups:

(1) Those reactions in which pyruvate, or a metabolic product of pyruvate, is reduced at the expense of NADH to give a reduced product such as lactate or ethanol. When this occurs, the conversion of glucose to final product proceeds with no *overall* reduction of NAD^+. All of the NADH is stoichiometrically reoxidized, because the number of molecules of oxidant (pyruvate) is equal to the number of molecules of substrate oxidized at the glyceraldehyde phosphate dehydrogenase reaction. In this situation, glycolysis is a self-contained process and requires no additional oxidation reagent such as molecular oxygen. It is, therefore, capable of operating under anaerobic conditions, and is the main metabolic pathway used for synthesizing ATP under such conditions.

(2) In the presence of oxygen many cells are able to oxidize NADH indirectly by the electron transport system. Under these conditions, pyruvate is not reduced and is therefore available for other reactions such as complete oxidation to carbon dioxide via the tricarboxylic acid cycle.

One feature of the glyceraldehyde phosphate dehydrogenase reaction is that the equilibrium is such that a high $NAD^+/NADH$ ratio is required in the cell to favour 3-phosphoglyceroyl phosphate formation (p. 26). The implication of this is that any other reaction coupled through NAD to glyceraldehyde phosphate dehydrogenase must favour NADH oxidation in order to maintain the high $NAD^+/NADH$ ratio. That this can take place effectively is shown by the high ratios of about 1000/1 found for $NAD^+/NADH$ in some cells.

Anaerobic glycolysis

One reaction for the reoxidation of glycolytically-produced NADH is that catalysed by lactate dehydrogenase:

$$
\begin{array}{c}
COO^- \\
| \\
C{=}O \\
| \\
CH_3
\end{array}
+ NADH + H^+ \; \rightleftharpoons \;
\begin{array}{c}
COO^- \\
| \\
HOCH \\
| \\
CH_3
\end{array}
+ NAD^+
$$

The equilibrium of this reaction is in favour of oxidation of NADH and formation of lactate, so it can couple effectively with the glyceraldehyde phosphate dehydrogenase reaction of glycolysis. In animals, the reaction is specific for the formation of L-lactate (as shown in the above formula) but in some bacteria, such as those used for cheese making, the product is D-lactate.

It has been known for many years that lactate is formed when muscles contract. The ability of muscles to carry out anaerobic glycolysis is of considerable survival value to the animal, since it allows for synthesis of the ATP required for contraction long before the physiological responses of the cardiovascular system can deliver sufficient oxygen to the tissues to allow complete oxidation of substrates to take place. The animal can, therefore, respond immediately to a threat from a predator or to some other stimulus. In fact, the muscles of mammals are specialized into two general types. The slow twitch ("red") fibres have a high mitochondrial content and are adapted to supply the ATP for contraction by aerobic metabolism. The fast twitch ("white") fibres contain fewer mitochondria but have high activities of phosphorylase, the glycolytic enzymes and lactate dehydrogenase. It is these fibres which are specialized for rapid anaerobic glycolysis, using glycogen as substrate and converting it to lactate. The white fibres have a poorer capillary system (and therefore oxygen supply) than the red fibres.

Lactic acid can accumulate in quite high concentrations in muscle during a heavy work load, and its presence may eventually lower the muscle pH to an extent that muscle function is impaired. Lactate is not usually further metabolized by muscle, but diffuses into the blood, where it is eventually carried to the liver and is there partly used for the resynthesis of glucose by gluconeogenesis (p. 62). The glucose may then be recycled back to the muscle to serve as substrate for glycogen resynthesis when the muscle is at rest. This process is known as the Cori cycle (figure 2.3).

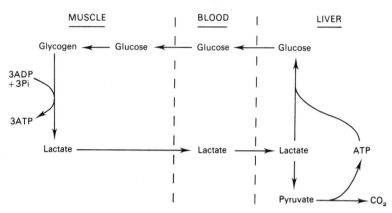

Figure 2.3   The Cori cycle. Some of the lactate produced by anaerobic glycolysis in muscle is converted back to glucose (and glycogen) by gluconeogenesis in the liver.

Other animal tissues are also able to carry out anaerobic glycolysis to give lactate. This ability is particularly important in mammalian red blood cells and in cells of the retina, which lack mitochondria and therefore cannot make use of oxygen for oxidation of substrates.

Ethanol is the product of anaerobic glycolysis ("fermentation") in yeast. It is formed in a sequence of two reactions in which pyruvate is first decarboxylated to acetaldehyde, which is then reduced with NADH to produce ethanol:

$$\underset{\substack{\textstyle | \\ \textstyle CH_3}}{\overset{\substack{\textstyle COO^- \\ \textstyle | \\ \textstyle C=O \\ \textstyle |}}{}} \xrightarrow{\text{pyruvate decarboxylase}} CO_2 + \underset{\substack{\textstyle | \\ \textstyle CH_3}}{\overset{\textstyle CHO}{}}$$

$$\underset{\substack{\textstyle | \\ \textstyle CH_3}}{\overset{\textstyle CHO}{}} + NADH + H^+ \underset{\text{dehydrogenase}}{\overset{\text{alcohol}}{\rightleftharpoons}} \underset{\substack{\textstyle | \\ \textstyle CH_3}}{\overset{\textstyle CH_2OH}{}} + NAD^+$$

The equilibrium of the dehydrogenase reaction favours NADH oxidation.

Tissues of higher plants may also produce ethanol when anaerobic conditions are encountered, as occurs in waterlogged ground, or during seed germination where oxygen penetration of the seed coat may be poor.

One advantage of ethanol as a product is that it does not affect the pH of the cell or its environment, as does an acidic product such as lactate. Yeast cells can tolerate quite high amounts of ethanol (during wine-making, the concentration may rise to about 12%). Such concentrations

are greatly in excess of those tolerated by mammals, since pharmacological effects of ethanol on the nervous system are apparent at concentrations of around 0.05 %. Lactate may be a preferred end-product of
anaerobic glycolysis in animals, because it can readily be recycled back to
carbohydrate, whereas, once decarboxylation of pyruvate to acetaldehyde
has taken place, the product can no longer be used for gluconeogenesis
(chapter 3).

Although lactate is the product of anaerobic glycolysis in many
animals, other products may be formed in invertebrates which live either
permanently or temporarily under anaerobic conditions. Thus, the parasitic tapeworms and roundworms live in the intestines of their hosts where
the oxygen tension is very low. The roundworm *Ascaris* produces a
number of different compounds during anaerobic metabolism, including
succinate, acetate, propionate and *n*-valerate. Figure 2.4 shows the main
pathway used by such organisms for the formation of succinate. One
feature of this pathway is that the pyruvate kinase reaction is bypassed.
Instead, phosphoenolpyruvate is carboxylated to give oxaloacetate in the
phosphoenolpyruvate carboxykinase reaction. Subsequent reduction of

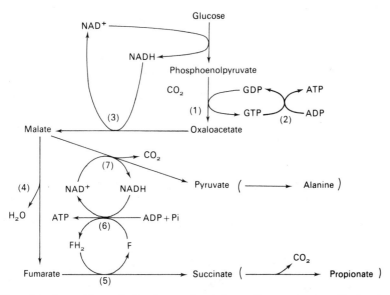

Figure 2.4   Anaerobic metabolism in some invertebrates. Key enzymes are: (1) phosphoenolpyruvate carboxykinase; (2) nucleoside diphosphate kinase; (3) malate dehydrogenase;
(4) fumarate hydratase; (5) succinate dehydrogenase; (6) part of the electron transport
system; (7) malate dehydrogenase (decarboxylating).

oxaloacetate to malate reoxidizes the NADH produced during glycolysis, and a further reduction step when fumarate is converted to succinate allows the concomitant oxidation of other substrates to take place. Part of the electron transport chain is used to transfer reducing equivalents from NADH to FAD, and additional ATP is synthesized at this step by oxidative phosphorylation.

Oysters are bivalve molluscs which can inhabit intertidal regions of the seashore. When the tide is high, the animals open their shells and extract nutrients and oxygen from the water. When the tide goes out, they close their shells together to prevent desiccation, and for the next few hours have to survive anaerobically. As with the parasitic worms, a major product of anaerobic metabolism in such molluscs is succinate.

The muscles of other invertebrates have yet another mechanism for reoxidizing NADH. They have arginine phosphate as phosphagen and, during muscle contraction, this is converted to arginine by the arginine kinase reaction. Pyruvate formed by glycolysis can react with the arginine to give octopine and reoxidize NADH:

(1)
$$\text{arginine-}P + \text{ADP} \underset{\text{arginine kinase}}{\rightleftharpoons} \text{ATP} + \text{arginine}$$

(2)
$$
\begin{array}{l}
\text{NH}_3^+ \\
| \\
\text{C=NH} \quad \text{COO}^- \\
| \qquad\qquad | \\
\text{NH} \quad +\text{C=O} + \text{NADH} + \text{H}^+ \\
| \qquad\qquad | \\
(\text{CH}_2)_3 \quad \text{CH}_3 \\
| \\
\text{CHNH}_3^+ \\
| \\
\text{COO}^- \\
\text{arginine} \quad \text{pyruvate}
\end{array}
\underset{\text{dehydrogenase}}{\overset{\text{octopine}}{\rightleftharpoons}}
\begin{array}{l}
\text{NH}_3^+ \\
| \\
\text{C=NH} \\
| \\
\text{NH} \\
| \\
(\text{CH}_2)_3 \quad \text{COO}^- \\
| \qquad\qquad | \\
\text{CH——N——CH} \\
| \quad\; | \quad\; | \\
\text{COO}^- \;\text{H} \;\; \text{CH}_3 \\
\text{octopine}
\end{array}
+ \text{NAD}^+ + \text{H}_2\text{O}
$$

Aerobic glycolysis

Under aerobic conditions, most cells are able to use molecular oxygen to oxidize NADH through the electron transport system. When this occurs, pyruvate is no longer required to act as oxidant for NADH, but is available either to be completely oxidized or to act as substrate for other reactions, such as fatty acid synthesis.

In the cells of eukaryotes, there is compartmentation between the reactions of glycolysis which occur in the cytosol (the soluble portion of the cytoplasm) and the reactions of the electron transport system (respiratory chain) which occur in the mitochondria, as the two systems are physically separated by the mitochondrial membranes. Mitochondria have two membranes, of which the inner membrane is selectively permeable to only a limited number of metabolites, and so controls the movement of substances in and out of the mitochondria. This membrane is not permeable to either NAD^+ or NADH, so there is no direct mechanism for the oxidation of NADH generated in the cytosol compartment by the mitochondrial electron transport system. Instead, there are a number of indirect systems for the transfer of reducing equivalents from cytosolic NADH into mitochondria. These are known as *shuttles* and involve the NADH-dependent reduction of a suitable substrate in the cytosol, followed by the transfer of reduced substrate into the mitochondrion. Here it is reoxidized by a second enzyme, so that the oxidation can be linked to the electron transport system. The oxidized substrate is then transported out of the mitochondrion to act as a carrier of further reducing equivalents from NADH.

Examples of such shuttles are shown in figure 2.5. The glycerol phosphate shuttle is particularly important in insect flight muscles which have a very high oxidative capacity. In these muscles, there is a plentiful oxygen supply because the tracheal system delivers oxygen directly to the fibres. Glycolysis in insect flight muscles is therefore geared closely to the complete oxidation of substrate, and the very active glycerol phosphate shuttle allows this to occur. A significant feature of the glycerol phosphate shuttle is that the two dehydrogenases are linked to different coenzymes. The cytosol glycerolphosphate dehydrogenase is specific for NAD, but the mitochondrial enzyme is linked to flavoprotein. Since the redox potential of the NAD^+/NADH couple is different from that of the oxidized/reduced flavin couple, the two dehydrogenase reactions have different equilibrium constants. For the mitochondrial enzyme, the equilibrium is much more in favour of the oxidation of glycerol phosphate than is the cytosol enzyme. This difference provides a mechanism for ensuring that the shuttle operates in the required direction only, and maintains the necessary high NAD^+/NADH ratio in the cytosol.

Another shuttle system for transporting reducing units into mitochondria is the malate/oxaloacetate shuttle shown in figure 2.5B. This system has been studied in mitochondria from mammalian liver and heart. The complexity of this shuttle is due to the impermeability of mitochondria to oxaloacetate. To transfer the oxaloacetate out of mitochondria, it is converted to a transportable product, aspartate, by a transamination between oxaloacetate and glutamate. The aspartate and

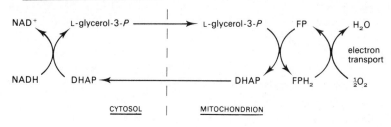

Figure 2.5 Shuttle systems for the transport of reducing equivalents from cytosol to mitochondrion.

2-oxoglutarate produced by this reaction are both transported out of the mitochondrion and then undergo a second transamination to regenerate oxaloacetate and glutamate in the cytosol.

In this scheme, both of the dehydrogenases use NAD as coenzyme, so the equilibrium constants of the reactions in the two compartments are identical. However, it is likely that the shuttle is unidirectional, because one of the transport systems is driven in the appropriate direction by an energy-linked reaction. The most likely site for this is the mitochondrial carrier which exchanges glutamate for aspartate across the membrane. This carrier probably exchanges glutamate ions plus protons from outside the mitochondria for aspartate ions inside the mitochondria. Since mitochondria generate a proton gradient across the membrane by energy-linked reactions associated with electron transport, this drives the amino-acid exchange in the required direction, and can account for the transport of reducing equivalents against an unfavourable NAD redox potential gradient.

Regulation of glycolysis

The relative importance of different glycolytic reactions in regulation, and the detailed mechanisms which operate, varies somewhat from one organism to another, and from one tissue to another within the same organism. There are, however, remarkable similarities in the pathway and its regulation in widely different species, which suggests that the optimum design of the pathway was approached long ago in evolution. Regulatory properties of enzymes have been evolved through acquired sensitivity to certain metabolites, which has presumably given the organisms selective advantages over competitors in being able to respond better to physiological stimuli.

Control reactions

The first control point in metabolism of carbohydrate is at the entry of substrate. The introduction of glycogen into metabolism at the phosphorylase reaction is subject to a complex series of controls (p. 121). The entry of monosaccharides may be controlled either by regulation of transport into the cell or by the rate of phosphorylation.

In many mammalian tissues, the transport of glucose into the cell is rate-limiting, and is controlled by a number of factors including hormones such as insulin (p. 177). In these tissues, the concentration of free glucose is low, because the capacity for phosphorylation by hexokinase usually exceeds the rate of transport into the cell. More rarely, the entry of glucose is not rate-limiting and then its metabolism may be controlled by the rate of phosphorylation. This is the situation in liver, where glucose is phosphorylated mainly by glucokinase. Because the K_m of glucokinase is high and similar to the concentrations of glucose in the liver cell, any increase in glucose concentration, such as occurs after intake of a carbohydrate-containing meal, results in an increase in the rate of phosphorylation. Such would not be the case for other (low K^m) hexokinases, since the glucose concentration would always be high enough to saturate the enzyme, so phosphorylation would proceed at maximum rate, irrespective of the substrate concentration.

As a general principle, regulatory enzymic reactions in the cell are usually found to be very far from their equilibrium position; that is, the mass-action ratios of their substrates and products are far away from the equilibrium ratios. These reactions occur at insufficient rates to equilibrate the reactants, and any change in their rate will change the rate at which substrate is converted to product, and the rate of the metabolic pathway as a whole. In contrast, non-regulatory enzymic reactions are catalysed by enzymes whose activity is high relative to the overall rate of the pathway, and whose reactants are therefore maintained at close to their equilibrium values. A change in the activity of such an enzyme would have little effect on the rate of the pathway as a whole, unless it was sufficiently large to decrease the activity to less than the flux through the pathway.

Three reactions of glycolysis are found to be far removed from equilibrium in nearly all organisms studied, and are therefore potential control points. These are the reactions catalysed by hexokinase, phosphofructokinase and pyruvate kinase.

The hexokinase reaction regulates the entry of glucose into metabolism in general, and not only into the glycolytic sequence. In many cells, hexokinase is inhibited by its reaction product, glucose 6-phosphate, so that, if there is a restriction in the rate of metabolism of hexose phosphates by any pathway, whether glycolysis, glycogen synthesis or pentose phosphate pathway, then accumulation of glucose 6-phosphate will prevent excessive phosphorylation of glucose.

Phosphofructokinase is the first enzyme which specifically commits substrate to glycolytic breakdown. It is subject to complex regulation by a number of factors (table 2.1), many of which affect the binding of ATP to a regulatory allosteric site on the enzyme. This site is separate from the active site and can be experimentally inactivated so that the enzyme is no longer inhibited by ATP, and yet retains its catalytic function.

Pyruvate kinase is also a regulatory enzyme. Its failure to approach equilibrium ensures that the intermediates of glycolysis do not become too depleted, and are maintained at a reasonable concentration, even when glycolysis is occurring at a slow rate. This is important in allowing the cell to respond rapidly to any increased requirements for glycolysis, and to provide substrate for synthetic reactions requiring glycolytic intermediates.

Regulation and energy metabolism

Since the most important function of glycolysis is to supply ATP for energy metabolism, it is reasonable to expect that the rate of glycolysis should be regulated in accordance with the energy requirements of the cell. Muscle is a good example of a tissue in which the rate of glycolysis is geared to the energy requirements. The relatively slow metabolic rate in resting muscle may be increased by more than one hundred times in contracting muscle, and this increase in rate is achieved within a few seconds. In such a short time, the main external influence on the muscle is nervous stimulation, since the circulation takes some time to deliver hormones to their site of action. The main regulatory influences on muscle at the early stage after onset of work are either a direct result of nervous stimulation or are caused by changes in concentrations of intermediates within the muscle which result from contraction.

Nervous stimulation of muscle causes release of calcium ions from the sarcoplasmic reticulum into the sarcoplasm. The contractile system responds to this increase by shortening, and the muscle contracts. Calcium ions also increase the breakdown of glycogen by activation of phosphorylase (p. 124) and thus make more substrate available for glycolysis. Perhaps surprisingly, phosphorylase seems to be the only glycolytic enzyme regulated by calcium ions.

As a result of muscle contraction, ATP is hydrolysed to ADP and orthophosphate. The activities of several key enzymes of glycolysis are affected by changes in the concentrations of adenine nucleotides and of orthophosphate, such that the rate of glycolysis tends to increase when concentrations of ATP fall, or when ADP and orthophosphate concentrations rise. Such effects therefore counteract the tendency for the ATP concentration to decrease by increasing the rate of glycolysis and hence the rate at which ADP is rephosphorylated.

Table 2.1 summarizes the effects of a number of metabolites ("effectors") on the main regulatory enzymes of glycolysis. Although all of these effects can be shown to occur when isolated enzymes are studied experimentally, the relative importance of the effects to the control of

Table 2.1   Some regulatory effects of metabolites on enzymes of glycolysis.

Enzyme	Positive effectors	Negative effectors
hexokinase (types I to III)		Glc-6-P
phosphofructokinase	AMP, ADP, Pi, Fru-6-P Fru-1,6-P_2, NH_4^+, K^+, cyclic AMP	ATP, citrate, creatine-P (muscle)
pyruvate kinase (liver)	AMP, Fru-1,6-P_2	ATP, alanine, citrate

glycolysis in living cells cannot be determined solely from a study of the properties of isolated enzymes. In addition, it is necessary to consider which of the effectors actually change in concentration in the tissue sufficiently to affect the rate of glycolysis when the muscle contracts. Thus measurements show a fall of only about 10 to 20% in ATP concentrations in contracting muscle, and this would be an insufficient signal to regulate glycolysis. The concentration of AMP on the other hand may increase to 2–3 times the resting value.

Such considerations lead to the conclusion that the effect of AMP on phosphofructokinase and other enzymes may play an important part in the regulation of glycolysis. Although AMP does not directly participate in most of the reactions in which ATP is used, its concentration is influenced by the relative concentrations of ATP and ADP in the cell, because of the presence of adenylate kinase which catalyses an equilibrium between the adenine nucleotides:

$$2\,ADP \rightleftharpoons ATP + AMP$$

The enzyme maintains the relative concentrations of the adenine nucleotides at close to equilibrium, so that any decrease in ATP concentration will lead to an increase in AMP concentration. Furthermore, at the relative concentrations of adenine nucleotides in the cell (high ATP, intermediate ADP, low AMP), it can be calculated that a fairly small fractional change in ATP concentration results in a much larger fractional change in AMP concentration. Since it is the proportional change in a signal which is most important in its ability to regulate enzyme activity, the concentration of AMP in the cell is a more sensitive signal of ATP concentration than is the ATP concentration itself. This use of AMP as a signal rather than ATP is of advantage because there are many reactions in the cell which depend on ATP as substrate, so it is essential to maintain a reasonably constant concentration of ATP. On the other hand, AMP is much less important in cellular reactions, so it is able to fluctuate over a wider range of concentrations and act as a regulatory signal.

A further refinement of the regulatory effects of adenine nucleotides on glycolysis is achieved in some tissues by a process known as substrate recycling. A good example of this occurs at the phosphorylation of fructose 6-phosphate. Muscles from a wide variety of organisms contain small but significant amounts of fructose 1,6-bisphosphatase which hydrolyses fructose 1,6-bisphosphate to fructose 6-phosphate. The combined action of this enzyme with phosphofructokinase can lead to recycling between the two substrates:

$$\text{Fru-6-}P + \text{ATP} \rightarrow \text{Fru-1,6-}P_2 \qquad \text{(phosphofructokinase)}$$
$$\text{Fru-1,6-}P_2 + \text{H}_2\text{O} \rightarrow \text{Fru-6-}P + \text{Pi} \quad \text{(fructose bisphosphatase)}$$

When both reactions occur at equal rates, there is no net phosphorylation of fructose 6-phosphate, but ATP is hydrolysed. However, the regulatory properties of the enzymes are such that both are never fully active at the same time. Fructose bisphosphatase is inhibited by AMP, and phosphofructokinase is activated by AMP. In resting muscle, the relatively low AMP concentration allows the phosphatase to be fairly active, whereas the kinase is largely inactive. Since the maximum activity of the phosphatase is only about 10% of the kinase, the net phosphorylation of

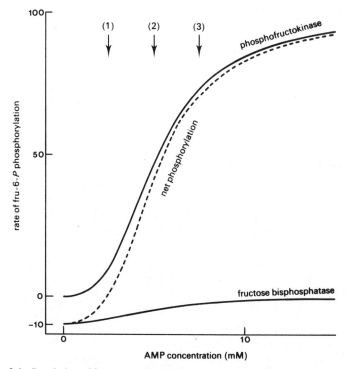

Figure 2.6 Regulation of fructose 6-phosphate phosphorylation through substrate recycling. The graph shows hypothetical values for the rate of phosphorylation, assuming that the maximum activity of fructose bisphosphatase is 10% of that of phosphofructokinase. At point (1), net phosphorylation is zero because the rate of phosphorylation is equal to that of dephosphorylation. At point (2), the AMP concentration has been increased two-fold, and the net rate of phosphorylation has increased to 50% of the maximum. At a three-fold increase in AMP (3), the net rate of phosphorylation is 75% of the maximum value (after Newsholme and Crabtree).

fructose 6-phosphate may be close to zero. This is shown graphically in figure 2.6.

The elevation in AMP which occurs during muscle contraction increases the net phosphorylation of fructose 6-phosphate both by activating phosphofructokinase and by inhibiting fructose bisphosphatase. The proportional increase in fructose 6-phosphate phosphorylation achieved by this mechanism is theoretically infinite, since the control rate is zero. Hence a moderate (2–3 fold) increase in AMP during contraction is an effective signal to increase the glycolytic rate. The cost to the organism of this regulatory mechanism is the small but continuous hydrolysis of ATP through the recycling of substrate.

A role for IMP in regulation of glycolysis in muscle has been proposed recently. This nucleotide is formed by AMP deaminase:

$$AMP \rightarrow IMP + NH_3$$

The rate of formation of IMP reflects the concentration of AMP in the cell. It has been found that IMP also affects regulatory enzymes and may be particularly important in activating phosphorylase.

Other regulatory influences

The effectors discussed so far are all involved in regulating glycolysis in its role in the energy metabolism of the cell. However, there are additional regulatory mechanisms which allow the glycolytic rate to respond to other factors. Thus citrate has an inhibitory effect on the phosphofructokinase reaction and acts as a signal for the operation of the tricarboxylic acid cycle. When there is ample substrate (pyruvate or fatty acids) for the tricarboxylic acid cycle, the citrate concentration is high and the rate of glycolysis is restricted through the regulatory effect of citrate. If the supply of substrate for the tricarboxylic acid cycle becomes limited, the citrate concentration falls; glycolysis is allowed to proceed at an increased rate, thus supplying more pyruvate as substrate for the tricarboxylic acid cycle. It is significant that both these pathways have a function in energy metabolism, so that, if sufficient ATP is being synthesized by complete oxidation of substrate in mitochondria, this should have a sparing effect on carbohydrate utilization. Indeed, this balance between carbohydrate utilization and oxidative metabolism has been known for many years as the *Pasteur effect*.

The main observation of the Pasteur effect is that in many different organisms the utilization of carbohydrates is inhibited in the presence of oxygen. The biochemical basis of the Pasteur effect is believed to lie at least partly in the regulation of the phosphofructokinase reaction. Increases in ATP and citrate concentrations, and decreases in AMP, ADP and orthophosphate will occur as a result of the operation of the tricarboxylic acid cycle under aerobic conditions, and these effectors will combine their effects to inhibit phosphofructokinase. This, in turn, will cause an increase in the concentrations of hexose phosphates until glucose is prevented from entering glycolysis by the inhibitory effect of glucose 6-phosphate on hexokinase. The Pasteur effect is of physiological advantage because oxidative metabolism uses substrates more economically than glycolysis, and does not lead to the accumulation of end-products (other than carbon dioxide). It is interesting to note that cells with no active tricarboxylic acid cycle, such as mammalian red blood cells, show no Pasteur effect.

Recent evidence has shown that at least two enzymes of glycolysis—phosphofructokinase and pyruvate kinase—exist in two interconvertible forms. In each case, one form is phosphorylated and the other form is not, and the two forms have different activities. Phosphorylation and dephosphorylation of these enzymes, therefore, provide an alternative mechanism for the regulation of carbohydrate metabolism, and may be one of the ways in which hormones act (chapter 10).

Pyruvate metabolism

In aerobic tissues, the breakdown of carbohydrate does not cease with the formation of pyruvate, but may continue until complete oxidation to carbon dioxide has been achieved. An outline of the pathway by which this oxidation is effected is shown in figure 2.7.

Pyruvate is first oxidized to acetyl-coenzyme A in a reaction catalysed by the pyruvate dehydrogenase complex. This reaction involves decarboxylation and oxidation of the substrate, followed by formation of the thioester, acetyl-CoA. This can then be completely oxidized by the reactions of the tricarboxylic acid cycle (also known as the citric acid cycle or the Krebs cycle). In this pathway, the acetyl-CoA is first condensed with oxaloacetate to form citrate, and in subsequent reactions the product is oxidized; two carbons are lost as carbon dioxide, and the oxaloacetate is regenerated to act as acceptor for synthesis of citrate from a further molecule of acetyl-CoA.

At the oxidation steps of the pathway, NAD^+ and flavin are reduced. The tricarboxylic acid cycle functions together with the respiratory chain, so that the reduced coenzymes are oxidized through the electron transport system, and some of the available energy is used to synthesize ATP from ADP and orthophosphate by the process of oxidative phosphoryl-

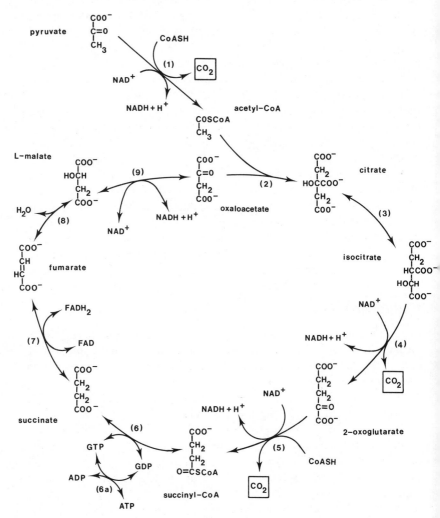

Figure 2.7 Pyruvate oxidation and the tricarboxylic acid cycle. The enzymes are: (1) pyruvate dehydrogenase; (2) citrate synthase; (3) aconitate hydratase; (4) isocitrate dehydrogenase; (5) 2-oxoglutarate dehydrogenase; (6) succinyl-CoA synthase; (6a) nucleoside diphosphate kinase; (7) succinate dehydrogenase; (8) fumarate hydratase; (9) malate dehydrogenase.

ation. The tricarboxylic acid cycle enzymes and the components of the respiratory chain are located within the mitochondria in eukaryotes.

The complete oxidation of pyruvate is summarized by the equation:

$$CH_3COCOOH + 2\tfrac{1}{2}O_2 \rightarrow 3CO_2 + 2H_2O$$

The three molecules of carbon dioxide are produced at three decarboxyl-ation reactions (pyruvate dehydrogenase, isocitrate dehydrogenase, and 2-oxoglutarate dehydrogenase). The uptake of oxygen is accounted for by the reduction of four NAD^+ molecules and of one FAD at the five dehydrogenase reactions, and the reoxidation of the reduced coenzymes by molecular oxygen through electron transport.

One of the main functions of the tricarboxylic acid cycle is to couple the oxidation of substrates to the synthesis of ATP. Complete oxidation of carbohydrate is much more effective in generating ATP than the partial breakdown of glucose to lactate or ethanol in anaerobic glycolysis. It may be recalled (p. 28) that anaerobic glycolysis yields two ATP molecules per glucose. However, the complete oxidation of glucose can yield some 36 ATP molecules from ADP. This figure is arrived at by assuming that each NADH is equivalent to 3 ATPs through oxidative phosphorylation, and that each reduced flavin can similarly give 2 ATPs. In this way, the four NADHs and one reduced FAD formed during pyruvate oxidation, together with the single GTP (synthesized by substrate phosphorylation at the succinyl-CoA synthase reaction) give an ATP equivalence of 15 per pyruvate. Glycolysis gives two pyruvate molecules per glucose, plus 2 ATPs from substrate-level phosphorylation, and a further 4 ATPs (from reduced flavin by linking the glyceraldehyde phosphate dehydrogenase reaction to electron transport through the glycerol phosphate shuttle). The sum of all these reactions gives the equivalent of 36 ATPs per glucose.

The function of the tricarboxylic acid cycle is not only to oxidize pyruvate. It is also the route for oxidation of acetyl-CoA produced from β-oxidation of fatty acids and of products of amino-acid degradation. It also has synthetic functions. Glucogenic amino acids can be converted to oxaloacetate via the tricarboxylic acid cycle, and can then be converted to carbohydrates by gluconeogenesis (p. 62); citrate is an intermediate in fatty-acid synthesis; and various amino acids, porphyrins, pyrimidines, etc., are all synthesized starting from intermediates of the cycle.

OTHER PATHWAYS OF
MONOSACCHARIDE METABOLISM

Interconversion of monosaccharides

The biological interconversion of monosaccharides fulfils two main functions: to introduce a variety of food carbohydrates into general metabolism, and to make available specific monosaccharides for synthesis of polysaccharides, nucleic acids and other cellular components.

Sugar interconversions can take place at three different levels: the free sugars, the sugar phosphates, and the nucleoside diphosphate sugars. Interconversion of free sugars is the least common type of reaction and usually involves either oxidation or reduction of the sugars. Interconversions of sugar phosphates are typically encountered where modification at carbons 1, 2 or 3 of the monosaccharide is to be made. The phosphate group is then normally attached to the highest-numbered carbon of the sugar molecule, so that the part of the molecule undergoing modification does not directly involve the phosphate group. Where modification of the sugar at carbon 4 or above is to take place, the nucleoside diphosphate derivative is used. Here the substituent is at carbon 1, again remote from the carbons involved in the interconversion reaction. Many reactions involving interconversion of nucleoside diphosphate sugars are on the pathway to polysaccharide synthesis. Since these derivatives are also normally required for synthesis of the glycosidic links in polysaccharides (chapters 7–9), the sugars are generated in the appropriate form for this function.

Interconversion of free monosaccharides

Many plants synthesize polyols by reduction of the corresponding aldose or ketose sugars, and use either NADH or NADPH as cofactor. The

46

polyols are then used to transport carbohydrate between different plant tissues. They also form a store of reducing power, as they can regenerate the reduced forms of coenzymes during their subsequent metabolism to ketose or aldose sugars.

In animals, reactions of free reducing sugars are fairly uncommon. One example occurs in mammalian seminal fluid, where the fructose present in high concentrations in semen is synthesized by reduction of D-glucose to D-glucitol, followed by reoxidation at C-2 to give D-fructose:

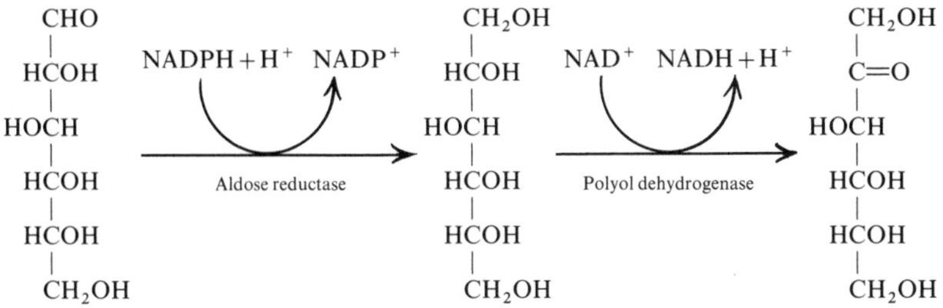

Although the reactions are reversible, fructose synthesis is favoured *in vivo* because of the high $NADPH/NADP^+$ ratio and low $NADH/NAD^+$ in cells.

Polyols are also found in the lens of the eye, where they arise from reduction of sugars by NADPH-linked dehydrogenases. In some diseases of defective carbohydrate metabolism, such as galactosemia and diabetes, where there are high concentrations of sugars in the blood, abnormally high concentrations of the corresponding polyols are found in the lens and can cause cataract formation and blindness.

Some microorganisms carry out the oxidation of free sugars by oxidase reactions in which molecular oxygen acts as the oxidizing reagent. Thus glucose oxidase catalyses the oxidation of D-glucose to D-glucono-1,5-lactone and hydrogen peroxide:

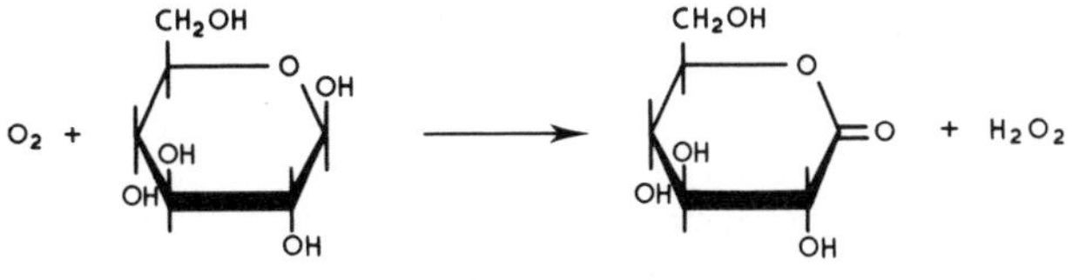

Purified glucose oxidase is used in many laboratories to estimate D-glucose. Hydrogen peroxide formed in the reaction is coupled to the oxidation of a suitable dye in the presence of peroxidase. The amount of coloured product formed can be measured and is proportional to the concentration of glucose in the unknown solution.

Glucose oxidase is also found in honey, where the hydrogen peroxide it produces acts as a preservative because it is toxic to microorganisms.

Interconversion of sugar phosphates

A common reaction in sugar metabolism is the interconversion of aldose phosphates and the corresponding ketose phosphates. Pairs of sugars interconverted by this type of reaction are listed in table 3.1. All of these reactions probably take place via an enediol intermediate according to the general equation:

$$
\underset{\text{ketose}}{
\begin{array}{c}
\text{OH} \\
| \\
\text{H--C--H} \\
| \\
\text{C=O} \\
| \\
\text{R}
\end{array}}
\rightleftharpoons
\left[
\begin{array}{cc}
\begin{array}{c}
\text{OH} \\
| \\
\text{H--C} + \text{H}^+ \\
|| \\
\text{C--O}^- \\
| \\
\text{R}
\end{array}
\rightleftharpoons
\begin{array}{c}
\text{OH} \\
| \\
\text{H--C} \\
|| \\
\text{C--OH} \\
| \\
\text{R}
\end{array}
\end{array}
\right]
\rightleftharpoons
\underset{\text{aldose}}{
\begin{array}{c}
\text{H--C=O} \\
| \\
\text{H--C--OH} \\
| \\
\text{R}
\end{array}}
$$

Although the reaction is shown as occurring with the acyclic forms of the sugars, it is possible that the ring forms of hexose and pentose phosphates participate in the reaction.

A rather similar reaction to the aldose/ketose interconversion takes place during the isomerization of D-ribulose 5-phosphate and D-xylulose 5-phosphate catalysed by ribulose-phosphate 3-epimerase:

$$
\underset{\text{ribulose-5-}P}{
\begin{array}{c}
\text{CH}_2\text{OH} \\
| \\
\text{C=O} \\
| \\
\text{HCOH} \\
| \\
\text{HCOH} \\
| \\
\text{CH}_2OP
\end{array}}
\rightleftharpoons
\left[
\begin{array}{ccc}
\begin{array}{c}
\text{CH}_2\text{OH} \\
| \\
\text{COH} \\
|| \\
\text{COH} \\
| \\
\text{HCOH} \\
| \\
\text{CH}_2OP
\end{array}
\rightleftharpoons
\begin{array}{c}
\text{CH}_2\text{OH} \\
| \\
\text{HCOH} \\
| \\
\text{C=O} \\
| \\
\text{HCOH} \\
| \\
\text{CH}_2OP
\end{array}
\rightleftharpoons
\text{HOC}
\begin{array}{c}
\text{CH}_2\text{OH} \\
| \\
\text{COH} \\
|| \\
\\
| \\
\text{HCOH} \\
| \\
\text{CH}_2OP
\end{array}
\end{array}
\right]
\rightleftharpoons \text{HOCH}
\underset{\text{xylulose-5-}P}{
\begin{array}{c}
\text{CH}_2\text{OH} \\
| \\
\text{C=O} \\
| \\
\\
| \\
\text{HCOH} \\
| \\
\text{CH}_2OP
\end{array}}
$$

Temporary transfer of the C-2 ketone group to the adjacent C-3 via an enediol intermediate destroys the chiral arrangement at C-3, so that the C-3 epimer can be produced when the ketone group is reformed at C-2. This reaction is part of the pentose phosphate pathway of metabolism (p. 52).

Table 3.1 Interconversions of aldose and ketose phosphates.

Enzyme	Aldose phosphate	Ketose phosphate	Metabolic role
triosephosphate isomerase	glyceraldehyde-3-P	dihydroxyacetone-P	glycolysis
glucosephosphate isomerase	glucose-6-P	fructose-6-P	glycolysis
mannosephosphate isomerase	mannose-6-P	fructose-6-P	mannose metabolism
ribosephosphate isomerase	ribose-5-P	ribulose-5-P	pentose-phosphate pathway

Other carbohydrate derivatives can also be made from sugar phosphates. The most common reaction for synthesis of amino sugars starts with the incorporation of an amino group at C-2 of fructose 6-phosphate, catalysed by glucosaminephosphate isomerase (glutamine-forming):

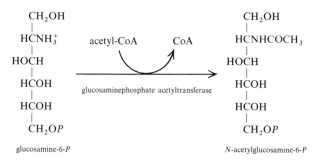

$$
\begin{array}{l}
\text{CH}_2\text{OH} \\
|\\
\text{C}{=}\text{O} \\
|\\
\text{HOCH} \\
|\\
\text{HCOH} \\
|\\
\text{HCOH} \\
|\\
\text{CH}_2\text{O}P
\end{array}
\;+\;
\begin{array}{l}
\text{CONH}_2 \\
|\\
(\text{CH}_2)_2 \\
|\\
\text{HCNH}_3^+ \\
|\\
\text{COO}^-
\end{array}
\;\rightleftharpoons\;
\begin{array}{l}
\text{CHO} \\
|\\
\text{HCNH}_3^+ \\
|\\
\text{HOCH} \\
|\\
\text{HCOH} \\
|\\
\text{HCOH} \\
|\\
\text{CH}_2\text{O}P
\end{array}
\;+\;
\begin{array}{l}
\text{COO}^- \\
|\\
(\text{CH}_2)_2 \\
|\\
\text{HCNH}_3^+ \\
|\\
\text{COO}^-
\end{array}
$$

fructose-6-P L-glutamine   glucosamine-6-P L-glutamate

Acetylation of the amino group can then occur:

$$
\begin{array}{l}
\text{CH}_2\text{OH} \\
|\\
\text{HCNH}_3^+ \\
|\\
\text{HOCH} \\
|\\
\text{HCOH} \\
|\\
\text{HCOH} \\
|\\
\text{CH}_2\text{O}P
\end{array}
\quad
\xrightarrow[\text{glucosaminephosphate acetyltransferase}]{\text{acetyl-CoA} \qquad \text{CoA}}
\quad
\begin{array}{l}
\text{CH}_2\text{OH} \\
|\\
\text{HCNHCOCH}_3 \\
|\\
\text{HOCH} \\
|\\
\text{HCOH} \\
|\\
\text{HCOH} \\
|\\
\text{CH}_2\text{O}P
\end{array}
$$

glucosamine-6-P N-acetylglucosamine-6-P

Oxidation of sugar phosphates can also take place. Glucose 6-phosphate dehydrogenase catalyses the oxidation of glucose

6-phosphate at C-1 to give 6-phospho-D-glucono-1,5-lactone. The lactone is then hydrolysed by a specific 6-phosphogluconolactonase to give the acyclic 6-phosphogluconate:

β-D-glucose-6-P   6-phospho-D-glucono-
                              1,5-lactone   6-phosphogluconate

Because the equilibrium of the lactonase reaction is far in favour of hydrolysis, the overall oxidation of glucose 6-phosphate to 6-phosphogluconate is physiologically irreversible.

Further oxidation of 6-phosphogluconate results in decarboxylation to give a pentose phosphate (ribulose 5-phosphate) in a reaction catalysed by phosphogluconate dehydrogenase. This reaction proceeds by oxidation at C-3 to give a ketone group β to the carboxylate group at C-1, and this favours the subsequent decarboxylation step. Carbon atom 1 of the hexose is lost as carbon dioxide:

6-phosphogluconate   ribulose-5-P

Interconversion of nucleoside diphosphate sugars

Table 3.2 lists the different types of chemical modification to monosaccharides that occur with the sugars as their nucleoside diphosphate derivatives. Because the sugars are substituted at the glycosidic carbon (C-1), the ring forms of the sugars are retained in these reactions.

One of the most common reactions is that of epimerization, such as occurs in the conversion of UDP-glucose to UDP-galactose catalysed by UDP-glucose 4-epimerase. The enzyme from yeast and some other sources has tightly-bound NAD as cofactor, whereas that from animal

Table 3.2 Sugar conversions involving nucleoside diphosphate sugars.

General reaction	Example	
	Enzyme	*Reaction*
epimerization	UDP-glucose 4-epimerase	UDP-glucose $\rightleftharpoons$ UDP-galactose
	UDP-arabinose 4-epimerase	UDP-L-arabinose $\rightleftharpoons$ UDP-D-xylose
oxidation	UDP-glucuronate decarboxylase	UDP-glucuronate $\rightarrow$ UDP-xylose
substitution	enoylpyruvate transferase	UDP-GlcNAc + PEP $\rightarrow$
		UDP-GlcNAc enoylpyruvate ether
rearrangement	UDP-glucuronate "cyclase"	UDP-glucuronate $\rightarrow$ UDP-apiose

tissues requires added NAD. The role of the NAD is to first oxidize the substrate at C-4 and thus destroy the chirality at that carbon. Subsequent reduction with the NADH produced in the first reaction can then give a product with a changed configuration at C-4:

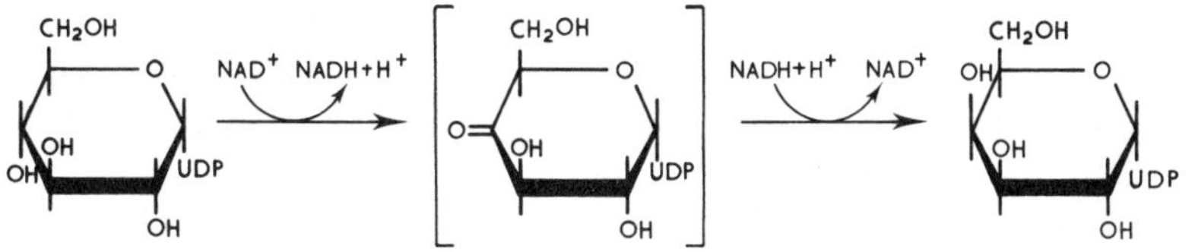

Uronic acids can be formed by oxidation of nucleoside diphosphate sugars at the carbon atom bearing the primary hydroxyl group. The oxidation of UDP-glucose occurs in two consecutive stages, involving reduction of two NAD^+ molecules, and with a C-6 aldehyde form of the sugar as an enzyme-bound intermediate:

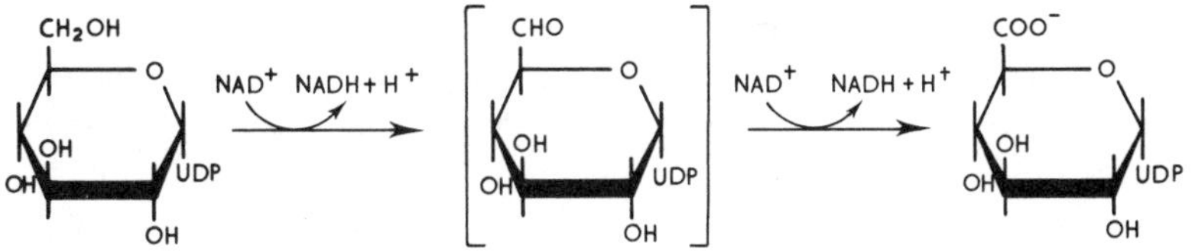

In plants, UDP-glucuronate is a precursor for pentoses and can be decarboxylated to give UDP-xylose. This reaction also requires NAD as cofactor, and the substrate is first oxidized at C-4, which provides a carbonyl group β to the carboxylate group and thus assists the decarboxylation reaction. After the decarboxylation has taken place, the C-4 ketone group is reduced, using the NADH formed at the initial oxidation reaction:

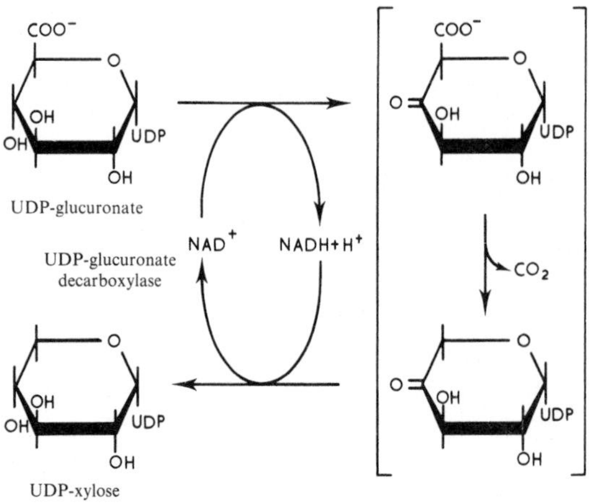

UDP-glucuronate

UDP-glucuronate decarboxylase

NAD^+ $NADH + H^+$

CO_2

UDP-xylose

The UDP-xylose formed in this reaction is in the pyranose form, because the hexose from which it is formed is a pyranose. The six-membered ring is also retained during subsequent polysaccharide synthesis, so that polysaccharides thus formed are composed of xylopyranose units.

Other reactions involving nucleoside diphosphate sugars include formation of branched chain sugars such as apiose (a component of plant glycosides) and streptose (part of the antibiotic streptomycin). UDP-N-acetyl muramic acid required for synthesis of bacterial cell walls is also synthesized as a nucleoside diphosphate sugar (p. 135).

The pentose phosphate pathway

Although glycolysis is the most common pathway for degradation of sugars, a number of alternative routes occur. The most common of these is the pentose phosphate pathway, which fulfils rather different functions from those of glycolysis.

The pentose phosphate pathway is also known as the hexose-monophosphate shunt, or phosphogluconate pathway, and consists of two distinct sections (figure 3.1). In the first section the oxidation of glucose 6-phosphate to ribulose 5-phosphate is carried out by the reactions described on pp. 49 to 50. This part of the pathway is physiologically irreversible. The second section of the pathway consists of a series of reversible reactions by which hexose and pentose phosphates are meta-

A Oxidative Section

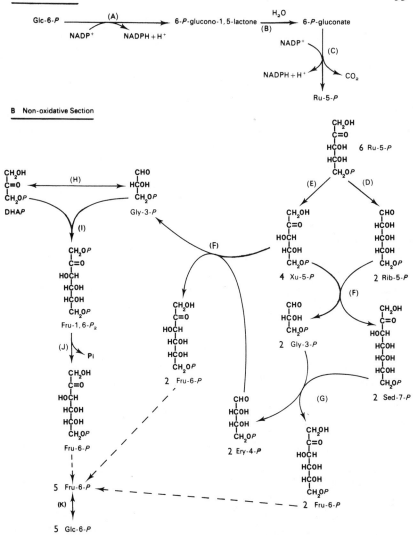

B Non-oxidative Section

Figure 3.1 The pentose phosphate pathway. The enzymes are: (A) glucose 6-phosphate dehydrogenase; (B) lactonase; (C) phosphogluconate dehydrogenase; (D) ribosephosphate isomerase; (E) ribulose 5-phosphate 3-epimerase; (F) transketolase; (G) transaldolase; (H) triosephosphate isomerase; (I) aldolase; (J) fructose bisphosphatase; (K) glucosephosphate isomerase. Abbreviations not previously defined are: Ru-5-P, ribulose 5-phosphate; Xu-5-P, xylulose 5-phosphate; Sed-7-P, sedoheptulose 7-phosphate; Gly-3-P, glyceraldehyde 3-phosphate; DHAP, dihydroxyacetone phosphate; Ery-4-P, erythrose 4-phosphate.

Note that for clarity the reversible reactions of the non-oxidative section have been shown to operate in the direction of hexose phosphate synthesis from pentose phosphate.

bolically interconverted. This reversible section of the pathway can lead either to hexose synthesis from pentoses, or to pentose synthesis from hexoses. It also provides metabolic links with three-, four-, and seven-carbon sugars.

Reactions of the non-oxidative section of the pathway are of two general types. The first type includes sugar interconversions of aldose and ketose phosphates, and epimerization reactions discussed earlier in this chapter. The second type of reaction involves transfer of two- and three-carbon sections of the sugar phosphate molecules from one sugar to another. Two-carbon transfers are catalysed by transketolase, and three-carbon transfers by transaldolase.

Transketolase has thiamin pyrophosphate bound covalently to the enzyme molecule, and this acts as cofactor. The reaction starts by transfer of a two-carbon unit from a suitable ketose phosphate onto the thiamin pyrophosphate of the enzyme to give an intermediate referred to as "active glycolaldehyde". The second stage of the reaction is virtually a reversal of the first stage—the two-carbon fragment is transferred from thiamin pyrophosphate onto an acceptor aldose phosphate. This re-generates the original form of the enzyme and yields a ketose phosphate with two carbons more than the acceptor aldose phosphate:

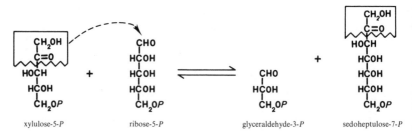

xylulose-5-P ribose-5-P glyceraldehyde-3-P sedoheptulose-7-P

Transketolase is relatively non-specific and can catalyse reactions between other pairs of sugar phosphates. In the pentose phosphate pathway, transketolase also catalyses a reaction between xylulose 5-phosphate and erythrose 4-phosphate to give fructose 6-phosphate and glyceraldehyde 3-phosphate.

The transaldolase reaction involves the transfer of a three-carbon unit from sedoheptulose 7-phosphate onto glyceraldehyde 3-phosphate to give erythrose 4-phosphate and fructose 6-phosphate. This reaction does not require a cofactor, but the three-carbon unit is transferred onto the enzyme molecule to form a Schiff's base complex with the amino group of a lysyl side-chain of the enzyme.

| sedoheptulose-7-P | glyceraldehyde-3-P | erythrose-4-P | fructose-6-P |

The oxidative and non-oxidative sections of the pentose-phosphate pathway can operate in different ways, depending on the organism or tissue and on the physiological circumstances. Thus the pathway has several different functions, and may fulfil one or more of these under a given set of conditions. These functions are:

(1) Provision of sugars for synthetic purposes. Pentoses are required for the synthesis of nucleotides and the nucleic acids. Erythrose 4-phosphate is used during synthesis of aromatic amino acids and other aromatic compounds in bacteria and plants. (Animals do not use erythrose 4-phosphate for this purpose and cannot synthesize aromatic compounds. They require preformed aromatic compounds, such as the amino acids tyrosine, phenylalanine, and tryptophan as essential components of the diet.) Inspection of figure 3.1 shows that pentose and erythrose phosphates can be derived from hexoses either by the non-oxidative section of the pentose phosphate pathway alone, or by the oxidative section in combination with some reactions of the non-oxidative section. Apparently both routes are used for this function.

(2) Reduction of $NADP^+$. The reduced form of NADP is specifically required for reductive biosynthetic reactions, such as synthesis of long-chain fatty acids from acetyl-CoA and reactions of steroid synthesis. These reactions are usually specific for NADPH as reductant rather than NADH, and this specificity is important in ensuring that the reactions proceed in the required direction. Thus the ratio of $NAD^+/NADH$ is very high in many cells (p. 30) to drive oxidative reactions such as glyceraldehyde phosphate dehydrogenase in the direction of substrate oxidation. On the other hand, the ratio of $NADP^+/NADPH$ is low, that is, much more strongly in favour of the reduced compound. This favours the reductive synthetic reactions. To maintain the NADP in the reduced form, secondary reactions are required to reduce the oxidized form of the coenzyme as it is formed.

This seems to be one of the main functions of the oxidative reactions of the pentose phosphate pathway. The two oxidative reactions are both $NADP^+$-specific and both have equilibria in favour of NADPH formation, and so favour a low $NADP^+/NADPH$ ratio.

There is good circumstantial evidence to support this role for the pentose phosphate pathway. Tissues such as lactating mammary gland, which synthesize large quantities of fatty acids, are also found to oxidize a considerable proportion of glucose through the oxidative pentose phosphate pathway, whereas other tissues (such as muscle) metabolize glucose almost exclusively by glycolysis.

In mammalian red blood cells, a proportion (10%) of glucose is metabolized through the pentose phosphate pathway to generate NADPH. This has a special function in red cells in that it maintains glutathione in the reduced form. The reduced glutathione is important in maintaining a number of proteins in the cell in an active state. It is also apparently involved in protecting the cell against haemolysis (leakage of haemoglobin and other cell components) during drug treatment.

Where large quantities of glucose are metabolized through the oxidative section of the pathway, the rate of pentose phosphate formation exceeds the cells' requirements for pentose. Under these conditions, pentose phosphates are recycled back to hexose phosphates via the non-oxidative section of the pathway. The pathway then operates for the overall oxidation of glucose:

$$6 \text{ glucose-6-}P + 12 \text{ NADP}^+ \rightarrow 6 \text{ pentose-5-}P + 6 \text{ CO}_2 + 12 \text{ NADPH} + 12 \text{ H}^+$$

$$6 \text{ pentose-5-}P \rightleftharpoons 5 \text{ glucose-6-}P$$

Sum: $\text{glucose-6-}P + 12 \text{ NADP}^+ \rightarrow 12 \text{ NADPH} + 12 \text{ H}^+ + 6 \text{ CO}_2$

(3) Complete oxidation of hexoses. In aerobic acetic acid bacteria, the pentose phosphate pathway is the major route for glucose degradation. In this case, the pathway is coupled to ATP synthesis as well as to synthetic reactions. Again, the pathway can operate in the cyclic mode shown above.

(4) Metabolism of non-hexose sugars. Pentoses and other sugars which may be present in food may be brought into the mainstream pathways of metabolism by the non-oxidative reactions of the pentose phosphate pathway.

(5) Photosynthesis. A modified pentose phosphate pathway is involved in assimilating carbon dioxide into carbohydrate during photosynthesis (chapter 4).

The regulation of the pentose phosphate pathway in many organisms is closely linked to the cells' requirements for NADPH. The most important regulatory enzyme of the pathway is glucose 6-phosphate dehydrogenase. This is inhibited by NADPH, and the inhibition is relieved by $NADP^+$, so that the rate of sugar metabolism through the pathway is controlled by the $NADPH/NADP^+$ ratio. This is in keeping with the proposed function of the pathway in maintaining NADPH for synthetic reactions. Although effects of NADPH and $NADP^+$ on glucose 6-phosphate dehydrogenase are not the only regulatory influences on the pathway, they seem to be the most universal effects and the best documented. Little is known of possible regulatory effects on the non-oxidative reactions of the pathway.

The Entner-Doudoroff pathway

Microorganisms use a number of different mechanisms for the breakdown of carbohydrates. These will not all be considered in detail here, but as an example the best-known of these, the Entner-Doudoroff pathway is shown in figure 3.2. This is the pathway by which bacteria of the *Pseudomonas* family degrade glucose.

The first step is the oxidation of glucose 6-phosphate to 6-phosphogluconate, as occurs in the oxidative section of the pentose phosphate pathway. The 6-phosphogluconate then undergoes a dehydration which results in oxidation at C-2 and reduction at C-3 to give 2-keto,3-deoxy 6-phosphogluconate. A specific aldolase acts on this to give pyruvate and glyceraldehyde 3-phosphate. The glyceraldehyde 3-phosphate is converted through the later reactions of glycolysis to give more pyruvate. Further metabolism of pyruvate in these aerobic organisms is by the tricarboxylic acid cycle.

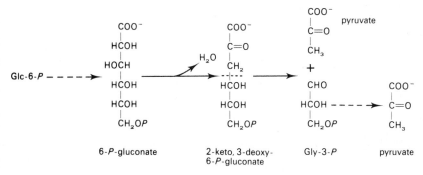

Figure 3.2 The Entner-Doudoroff pathway of carbohydrate metabolism in *Pseudomonas*.

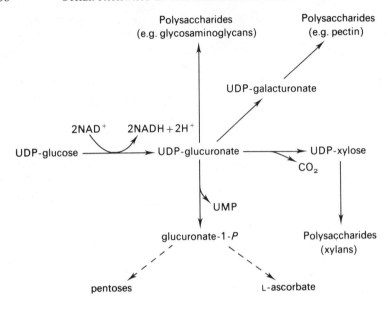

Figure 3.3   Metabolism of UDP-D-glucuronate.

Metabolism of glucuronate

Figure 3.3 summarizes the main ways in which glucuronate is metabolized. Glucuronate is synthesized from glucose as its UDP derivative (p. 51), and can then either give polysaccharides directly or can undergo modification to other sugars and then give polysaccharides. Alternatively, after hydrolysis to glucuronate 1-phosphate and then free glucuronate, it can give a range of different monosaccharide derivatives including ascorbic acid (vitamin C).

The initial step in the metabolism of free D-glucuronate is its reduction at C-1 to give L-gulonate (figure 3.4). This product has a different configurational carbon from that of the substrate, and belongs to the L-series of sugars. D-Glucuronate is numbered from the aldehyde group at C-1, so that the carboxylate group is at C-6. However, when the aldehyde group at C-1 is reduced to a hydroxyl group, as in L-gulonate formation, the carboxylate group (originally designated C-6) becomes the main functional group, so the new compound must be renumbered with this group designated C-1. For nomenclature purposes, the whole molecule is therefore inverted. One of the results of this is that a new chiral carbon becomes the configurational carbon. Thus the highest numbered chiral carbon in gulonate is at the "new" C-5 (C-2 of D-glucuronate). Since this is in the L-configuration, the sugar belongs to the L-series. The configuration at the other chiral carbons corresponds to that of L-gulonate.

L-Gulonate can be metabolized in one of two ways. It can either give L-ascorbate (see next section), or it can undergo oxidation and decarboxylation to give pentoses. The latter pathway is present in mammals, but may not have an essential function since individuals lacking one of the enzymes of this pathway survive without any apparent ill-effects. Indeed, such an enzymic defect can only be recognized because of the presence of L-xylulose (one of the intermediates of the pathway) in the urine.

L-Ascorbate (vitamin C)

L-Ascorbate is an essential compound for all vertebrates, and also probably for animals of other groups, including the insects. Many

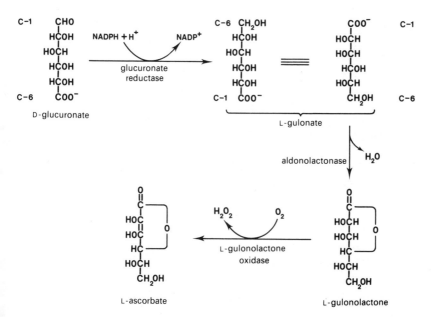

Figure 3.4   Conversion of D-glucuronate to L-ascorbate.

vertebrates are able to synthesize ascorbate in sufficient quantities to supply their own needs. This they do by oxidation of L-gulono-1,5-lactone by the reactions shown in figure 3.4. The enzymes of this pathway are found either in the liver (in mammals and some birds) or in the kidney (in amphibians and reptiles). For these groups, ascorbate is not a vitamin, as it is not required in the diet.

Other animals do not have the ability to synthesize ascorbate, and must therefore obtain it in their food. For them, ascorbate is a vitamin. Animals that require ascorbate in their diet include man and other primates, the guinea pig, flying mammals (bats) and some birds.

When humans feed on a diet lacking vitamin C, the ascorbate is gradually lost from the tissues until after about four months the deficiency symptoms of scurvy appear. Scurvy is characterized by haemorrhages, poor wound healing, loosening of the teeth, and other symptoms of defects in connective-tissue synthesis. Guinea pigs develop vitamin C deficiency after only about three weeks on a deficient diet.

Scurvy is relieved by a suitable diet containing ascorbate. Most plant foods contain some vitamin C, citrus fruits and green vegetables being particularly good sources. Potatoes are also valuable because, although they contain a lower concentration of the vitamin, often fairly large quantities of potatoes are consumed in the diet. The process of cooking has an adverse effect on the vitamin C content of vegetables, partly because some leaches out into the cooking water and is discarded, and partly because some is oxidized irreversibly by atmospheric oxygen.

The recommended daily intake of vitamin C varies (according to the authority making the recommendation) from 20 to 70 mg per day for an adult person. Amounts of this quantity are sufficient to prevent development of the symptoms of scurvy. However, there are also more controversial claims that much larger intakes of vitamin C, in the range of 1 to 5 grams per day, have beneficial effects in protection against the common cold, influenza and perhaps heart disease, and also promote wound healing. This view is advocated by Pauling (see references) but is not generally accepted by all nutritionists.

Several different functions have been proposed for the role of ascorbate in tissues. It is required for the hydroxylation of lysine and proline during the synthesis of collagen. Lack of vitamin C adversely affects connective tissues by interfering with this process. However, the actual molecular mechanism by which the ascorbate participates in this reaction is not known. Ascorbate also acts as an antioxidant because of its ready conversion to dehydroascorbate:

L-ascorbate   2-dehydro-L-ascorbate

Ascorbate may be particularly important for the survival of land-living animals, because they are exposed to high concentrations of oxygen. Oxygen can be damaging to tissues by virtue of reactions which give the toxic superoxide anion O_2^-. Ascorbate has been suggested to act as a scavenger of superoxide, and can thus protect tissues against its toxic effects.

Myo-inositol

One of the major groups of phospholipids is the phosphoinositides which contain *myo*-inositol. The most common of these is phosphatidylinositol:

R_1 and R_2 are fatty acids

This has a role, along with other groups of phospholipids, as a component of biological membranes. In the plasma membrane, inositol may have a particular function in cell regulation. The turnover of phosphatidylinositol is increased when mammalian cells are treated with certain hormones or neurotransmitters. When this occurs, the calcium-ion concentration in the cytosol of the cells is elevated. It has been suggested by Michell that phosphatidylinositol turnover in some way triggers the transport of calcium ions through the membrane, or the release of calcium ions from an intracellular site. The calcium then acts as a second messenger in regulating specific reactions within the cell (p. 179).

Most organisms can synthesize inositol as the phosphate ester by a cyclization reaction with glucose 6-phosphate as substrate:

myo-inositol-1-*P*

C-6 of the glucose molecule becomes C-1 of *myo*-inositol.

In some plant seeds, *myo*-inositol is stored as its hexaphosphate ester (phytic acid) in which all of the hydroxyl groups are substituted with orthophosphate. During germination, the phytic-acid stores are drawn on as a source of phosphate and carbohydrate for the growing plant.

Gluconeogenesis

Gluconeogenesis is a process by which carbohydrates can be synthesized from non-carbohydrate precursors in a series of reactions which virtually reverse glycolysis.

Many of the reactions of gluconeogenesis are identical to those of glycolysis, although, of course, the overall directions of the two pathways are opposite to each other (figure 3.5). Indeed, in tissues such as liver, many of the same enzymes are involved in both glycolysis and gluconeogenesis, and the direction of carbohydrate metabolism depends on the physiological conditions and the activities of certain key regulatory enzymes.

Certain enzymic reactions of glycolysis are found to be physiologically irreversible in all organisms (chapter 2). These are the reactions catalysed by phosphofructokinase, pyruvate kinase, and hexokinase. The other reactions of glycolysis are physiologically reversible and therefore can

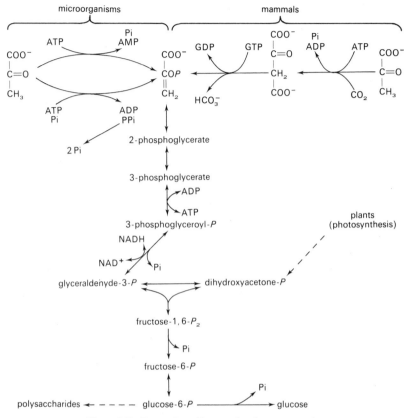

Figure 3.5   Formation of hexoses by gluconeogenesis.

operate in either direction. The ability of an organism or tissue to carry out gluconeogenesis therefore depends on whether it can bypass the irreversible reactions of glycolysis by alternative steps.

Gluconeogenesis is much more restricted in its tissue distribution than is glycolysis. Thus, in mammals, only liver and kidney have significant gluconeogenic capacities, whereas other tissues such as muscle, brain and adipose tissue have all of the glycolytic enzymes but lack one or more of the enzymes required for gluconeogenesis.

The conversion of pyruvate to phosphoenolpyruvate is the first requirement for gluconeogenesis from some substrates. Some bacteria and plants are able to do this by the pyruvate, water dikinase reaction:

$$\text{pyruvate} + \text{ATP} + \text{H}_2\text{O} \rightarrow \text{phosphoenolpyruvate} + \text{AMP} + \text{Pi}$$

This reaction involves the removal of *two* of the phosphate groups from ATP. Since the hydrolysis of both phosphate groups is considerably exergonic, the overall reaction can proceed in the direction of phosphoenolpyruvate formation. The reformation of ATP from AMP is equivalent to two ATP-ADP conversions, so to reverse the pyruvate kinase reaction (where one ATP is synthesized from ADP) the equivalent of two ATPs is used. Another reaction of this type found in bacteria is the pyruvate, phosphate dikinase reaction which also results in phosphoenolpyruvate synthesis:

$$\text{pyruvate} + \text{ATP} + \text{Pi} \rightarrow \text{phosphoenolpyruvate} + \text{ADP} + \text{PPi}$$

The inorganic pyrophosphate is then hydrolysed by pyrophosphatase, and product formation is thus favoured.

In mammals and probably other animals, a different process is used for phosphoenolpyruvate formation. Pyruvate is first carboxylated to oxaloacetate in the pyruvate carboxylase reaction, and the oxaloacetate is converted to phosphoenolpyruvate by phosphoenolpyruvate carboxykinase:

$$\text{pyruvate} + \text{HCO}_3^- + \text{ATP} \rightarrow \text{oxaloacetate} + \text{ADP} + \text{Pi}$$
$$\text{oxaloacetate} + \text{GTP} \rightarrow \text{phosphoenolpyruvate} + \text{GDP}$$

This mechanism for phosphoenolpyruvate formation, like that of the pyruvate, water dikinase reaction, uses the equivalent of two ATPs, since GDP can be converted back to GTP at the expense of ATP by nucleoside diphosphate kinase.

In some animals (e.g. rabbits) both of these enzymes of phosphoenolpyruvate formation are in the mitochondria, and the phosphoenolpyruvate is transported out for further metabolism. However, in other animals (e.g. rats), the pyruvate carboxylase is in the mitochondria, and the phosphoenolpyruvate carboxykinase is in the cytosol. Since the intermediate (oxaloacetate) which links these two reactions is not normally transported through mitochondrial membranes, it is first converted to a transportable intermediate, malate, to be exported from the mitochondria (figure 3.6). In the cytosol, the malate is converted back to oxaloacetate by malate dehydrogenase, and this reaction also generates NADH from NAD^+. The NADH is required in gluconeogenesis for reduction of substrate at the glyceraldehyde phosphate dehydrogenase reaction, so the process of malate transport out of mitochondria supplies both the substrate and the reducing equivalents for gluconeogenesis.

The second unique reaction of gluconeogenesis is the hydrolysis of

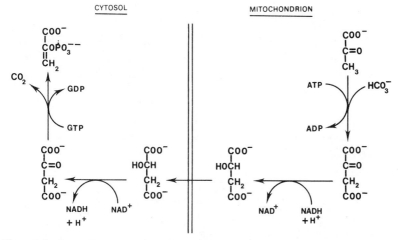

Figure 3.6 Conversion of pyruvate to phosphoenolpyruvate, and transport of substrate out of mitochondria during gluconeogenesis in rat liver.

fructose bisphosphate to give fructose 6-phosphate. The fructose bisphosphatase reaction opposes that of the phosphofructokinase reaction of glycolysis, and both enzymes are present together in tissues such as liver. If both enzymes were to be active at the same time, they would operate as a "futile cycle" to recycle substrate between fructose 6-phosphate and fructose biphosphate (p. 40). However, the enzymes are regulated by AMP so that, at high AMP concentrations, phosphofructokinase is active and hence glycolysis is favoured, whereas, at low AMP concentrations, phosphofructokinase becomes less active while fructose bisphosphatase is activated to favour gluconeogenesis.

The third irreversible reaction of glycolysis is the hexokinase reaction, and glucose 6-phosphate formed during gluconeogenesis can be converted to glucose by glucose 6-phosphatase. This enzyme is particularly important in mammalian liver, because it has a role in maintaining blood glucose concentrations. The reaction is not specific to gluconeogenesis, but is also involved in the conversion of glycogen to glucose.

In many organisms, the hexose phosphates produced by gluconeogenesis do not give free glucose but are used for synthesis of polysaccharides (e.g. in microorganisms) or sucrose (in many plants). The activity of glucose 6-phosphatase cannot therefore be regarded as an essential reaction of gluconeogenesis in all tissues, but only occurs where free glucose is the end-product.

Substrates for gluconeogenesis

Many compounds are used as substrates for gluconeogenesis. Some substrates are converted to gluconeogenic substrates through quite simple processes. Lactate is a quantitatively-important substrate for gluconeogenesis in the liver, and is produced by anaerobic glycolysis in extrahepatic tissues such as red blood cells and exercising muscle. Lactate is readily converted to pyruvate by lactate dehydrogenase.

Many amino acids are also good gluconeogenic precursors. Thus, transamination of alanine gives pyruvate, and of aspartate gives oxaloacetate, and both of these products are used for gluconeogenesis. Some other amino acids give intermediates of the tricarboxylic acid cycle by several-step processes, and can be converted to oxaloacetate in this way. In mammals, muscle proteins are an important source of gluconeogenic substrate, especially during starvation. They are hydrolysed to amino acids, some of which are converted to alanine in the muscle and are transported to the liver in this form. Glutamine is also produced during protein breakdown in muscle, and can be used by the kidneys.

Compounds such as fatty acids which give acetyl-CoA as an intermediate in their degradation, cannot be converted to carbohydrate in higher animals. This is because the pyruvate dehydrogenase reaction is irreversible, and there is no available mechanism for synthesizing three or four carbon gluconeogenic precursors from acetate. However, some microorganisms and plants are able to convert acetate (and therefore fatty acids) to carbohydrates because they have an additional pathway available. This is the glyoxylate bypass (p. 67).

In mammals, gluconeogenesis occurs under all physiological conditions, but becomes particularly important during starvation. Carbohydrate stored as glycogen in the liver is depleted relatively quickly in the absence of a dietary supply of carbohydrate, so that little is left after about 48 hours. The animal then depends heavily on its stored fat reserves as an energy source. Some carbohydrate is still required, however, for certain tissues such as the brain and red blood cells which use glucose as their main fuel. During starvation, the glucose concentration in the blood is maintained at close to the normal concentration (about 5 mM in many animals) to supply these essential tissues.

In addition to amino acids and lactate, glycerol can also provide gluconeogenic substrate during starvation. Glycerol is released during the hydrolysis of triglycerides in adipose tissue, and is not further metabolized there because adipose tissue lacks the glycerol kinase necessary to phosphorylate it. Instead, the glycerol passes to the liver, where it is phosphorylated, oxidized to dihydroxyacetone phosphate, and is hence converted to hexose:

$$\text{glycerol} + \text{ATP} \xrightarrow{\text{glycerol kinase}} \text{L-glycerol } 3\text{-}P + \text{ADP}$$

$$\text{L-glycerol } 3\text{-}P + \text{NAD}^+ \xrightarrow{\text{glycerol phosphate dehydrogenase}} \text{dihydroxyacetone-}P + \text{NADH} + \text{H}^+$$

During photosynthesis in green plants, triose phosphates are generated inside the chloroplasts and are then transported to the cytosol for further metabolism (p. 79). A major pathway in many plants is the conversion of such triose phosphates to sucrose, which requires part of the gluconeogenesis pathway. Gluconeogenesis also occurs in microorganisms grown on non-carbohydrate nutrients.

The glyoxylate bypass

The main function of the glyoxylate bypass is to generate four-carbon intermediates from two-carbon compounds such as acetate. It provides a link whereby two-carbon compounds and their precursors, particularly long-chain fatty acids, can be used as substrates for synthesis of carbohydrates and many other compounds essential to the cell. The glyoxylate bypass is found in some microorganisms and plants, but does not occur in higher animals.

The glyoxylate bypass pathway includes some enzymic reactions of the tricarboxylic acid cycle in combination with two additional enzymes— isocitrate lyase and malate synthase:

isocitrate

$$
\begin{array}{c}
\text{COO}^- \\
| \\
\text{CH}_2 \\
| \\
\text{HCCOO}^- \\
| \\
\text{HOCH} \\
| \\
\text{COO}^-
\end{array}
\xrightarrow{\text{isocitrate lyase}}
\begin{array}{c}
\text{COO}^- \\
| \\
\text{CH}_2 \quad \text{succinate} \\
| \\
\text{CH}_2 \\
| \\
\text{COO}^- \\
+ \\
\text{CHO} \\
| \quad \text{glyoxylate} \\
\text{COO}^-
\end{array}
$$

glyoxylate
+
acetyl-CoA

$$
\begin{array}{c}
\text{COO}^- \\
| \\
\text{CHO} \\
+ \\
\text{CH}_3 \\
| \\
\text{COSCoA}
\end{array}
\xrightarrow{\text{malate synthase}}
\begin{array}{c}
\text{COO}^- \\
| \\
\text{HOCH} \quad + \text{CoASH} \\
| \\
\text{CH}_2 \\
| \\
\text{COO}^-
\end{array}
$$

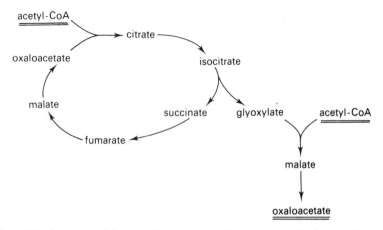

Figure 3.7   Operation of the glyoxylate bypass to show net synthesis of one molecule of oxaloacetate from two molecules of acetyl-CoA.

The significance of the isocitrate lyase reaction is that it bypasses the reactions of the tricarboxylic acid cycle (isocitrate dehydrogenase and 2-oxoglutarate dehydrogenase) at which carbons are lost as carbon dioxide. Instead, the two carbons are retained as glyoxylate, which can then react with acetyl-CoA to give malate.

The overall operation of the glyoxylate bypass is shown in figure 3.7. The net result of the pathway is that two molecules of acetyl-CoA are used (one at the citrate synthase step and one at malate synthase) and the product is succinate, which can be converted to oxaloacetate by reactions of the tricarboxylic acid cycle. Oxaloacetate can then act as a precursor for the synthesis of many essential cell components, including carbohydrates and some amino acids.

The enzymes of the glyoxylate bypass are only found in organisms for which acetate, or other one- or two-carbon compounds, is the main carbon source. Thus, a microorganism grown on acetate will have both isocitrate lyase and malate synthase in significant amounts, but these enzymes are not induced if the same microorganism is grown on other substrates such as glucose. Similarly, in plants, the enzymes are only found in tissues which require them. Triglycerides form the major reserves of certain types of "oleaginous" seeds such as the castor bean. When the seeds germinate, triglycerides are converted to the carbohydrates required by the growing plant. (Plants generally have a high carbohydrate content, partly because of their thick cell walls which are mainly carbohydrate.)

Plant seedlings of this type which use the glyoxylate bypass, have specialized organelles known as *glyoxysomes* in which the reaction of the glyoxylate bypass are segregated from other parts of the cell. Such organelles oxidize triglycerides and convert them to succinate. The succinate is then transported to mitochondria, where it is oxidized to oxaloacetate. Finally, the oxaloacetate can be converted to carbohydrate by gluconeogenesis in the cytosol.

CHAPTER FOUR

PHOTOSYNTHESIS

Nearly all the organic compounds used by living organisms are ultimately derived from carbon dioxide by plants and other photosynthetic organisms. In photosynthesis, light energy is used in the reduction of carbon dioxide to give firstly carbohydrates, and from these all of the other organic compounds required by cells.

It has been estimated that about 10^{11} tons of carbon dioxide are assimilated each year by photosynthesis. Eventually the carbon is returned to the atmosphere as plants, animals and microorganisms oxidize the organic compounds to recover some of the potential chemical energy stored in them.

The biochemical process of photosynthesis involves two distinct reaction sequences, known as the *light reaction* and the *dark reaction*. In the cell, both sequences occur together, both are required for photosynthesis, and one sequence is dependent on the other. However, because the reaction sequences can be separated experimentally, and because they involve different types of chemical reaction, it is convenient to consider them separately. In the light reaction, the energy from sunlight is used to reduce $NADP^+$ to NADPH, and to phosphorylate ADP to ATP. In the dark reaction, carbon dioxide is assimilated, and the NADPH and ATP produced in the light reaction are used to drive the reductive endergonic synthesis of carbohydrates.

Photosynthesis in green plants is carried out solely in the chloroplasts. These are subcellular organelles about 5 to $10\,\mu m$ long; that is, rather larger than mitochondria. Like mitochondria, they are surrounded by a double membrane which presents a permeability barrier to the movement of substrates. Inside the chloroplast are the pigmented *thylakoids* which consist of flattened sacs, the interiors of which are bounded by membranes. The thylakoids are generally arranged in stacks known as *grana* (figure 4.1). The complete machinery for the light reactions of photosynthesis is contained within the thylakoids. The dark reactions of photosynthesis occur in the largely soluble fraction or *stroma* of the chloroplast.

The light reaction

The first requirement for any photosynthetic system is a pigment capable of absorbing light energy. In plants, the main pigments are the green chlorophylls *a* and *b*, but in addition, secondary pigments such as carotenoids also occur. The pigments are arranged tightly packed together and associated with proteins and glycolipids in the thylakoids.

Photons of light can be absorbed by any of the pigment molecules in the thylakoids. During the absorption process, the energy of the photon is transferred to the pigment and can cause a ground-state electron of the molecule to be transferred to a higher-energy orbital. When this occurs, the pigment molecule is said to be *in an excited state*. Molecules in the excited state are unstable and have a lifetime of only about 10^{-9} second. Although such molecules can lose their energy by emitting a secondary photon (i.e. fluorescence) and thus return to the ground state, in the closely-packed pigment system of the thylakoids the energy is usually lost by transfer to an adjacent pigment molecule. Such energy transfers are

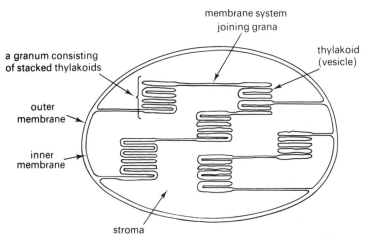

Figure 4.1 Diagram of chloroplast structure. The light reactions of photosynthesis occur in the thylakoids and the dark reactions in the stroma.

permitted, provided that the receiving molecule can absorb light of the same or a longer wavelength than the original molecule. (Photons of long wavelengths have lower energies than those of short wavelengths.) Eventually, by energy-transfer reactions between pigment molecules, a pair of specialized chlorophyll *a* molecules at the "trapping centre" become excited.

The pigments and other components of the thylakoids are organized into groups of "photosynthetic units" containing about 200 to 300 chlorophyll molecules and a number of secondary pigment molecules, but with a single trapping centre. Absorption of a photon by any pigment of the photosynthetic unit results in the energy being transferred to the trapping centre. Photons from almost any part of the visible spectrum (400–700 nm) may be absorbed and their energy used for photosynthesis. In plants (but not photosynthetic bacteria) there are two different types of

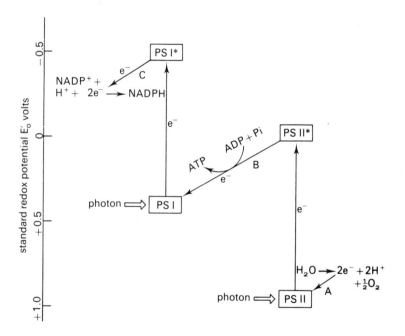

Figure 4.2 Electron transport during photosynthesis. Electrons tend to flow towards carriers with the more positive redox potentials. The exceptions are at the two photosystems, where input of energy in the form of a photon of light excites an electron at the trapping centre, increases its tendency to leave the molecule, and thus produces a molecule with a more negative potential.

* represents the excited PS state.

photosynthetic unit known as *photosystem I* (PS I) and *photosystem II* (PS II). These occupy different positions in the chain of electron carriers which link electron removal from water (oxidation) to reduction of $NADP^+$ (see below).

The next step of the reaction occurs when the excited electron of the trapping centre is used to reduce the oxidized component of an electron transport chain. Chloroplasts, like mitochondria, contain a series of electron carriers linked together as an electron-transport system. Each carrier can exist in either an oxidized or reduced form, and the components are arranged in sequence such that the reduced form of one carrier will pass on electrons to the oxidized form of the next carrier. (The first carrier becomes oxidized, and the second reduced.) The components of an electron transport system have different tendencies to lose electrons, that is, they have different standard redox potentials (E_0'). They are normally arranged in order of their redox potentials so that electrons tend to move "downhill" towards the carrier of most positive potential. Energy is lost from the system in this process, but some can be recovered by coupling electron transport to other reactions, such as ATP synthesis as in mitochondria. In photosynthesis, the *overall* electron flow is in the "wrong" direction: from water oxidation ($E_0' + 0.8V$) to $NADP^+$ reduction ($E_0' - 0.3V$). Energy has therefore to be put into the system, and this is done at two points corresponding to photosystems I and II. The transport chain for electrons in photosynthesis is shown in figure 4.2.

The chain starts with the oxidation of water by a strongly positive redox carrier:

$$H_2O \rightarrow \tfrac{1}{2}O_2 + 2e^- + 2H^+$$
$$\text{carrier} + 2e^- \rightarrow \text{carrier}^{--}$$

Electrons then flow "downhill" in section A of the chain as far as photosystem II, where they receive their first boost to the next section of the chain, which is at a less positive redox potential. When the trapping centre chlorophyll molecule is excited by light, an electron is raised to a higher-energy state as discussed above. This increases the tendency of the electron to leave the molecule. In other words, the molecule in the excited state is a much better electron donor (reducing agent) than the same molecule in the ground state. The electron is therefore donated from the excited PS II trapping-centre chlorophyll to the first component of section B of the electron transport chain. This leaves the chlorophyll with a positive charge which can be replaced by an electron from section A of the chain.

Electrons now move "downhill" in section B of the chain, and some of the energy available is coupled to ATP synthesis. The electrons then receive a second boost at photosystem I to reduce the most electro-negative components of section C of the chain. Here the electrons are passed on to reduce $NADP^+$ to NADPH.

As noted above, ATP is synthesized from ADP during the electron transport process. The stoichiometry of this coupling has not been firmly established, but either one or two ATPs are synthesized for each pair of electrons passing down the chain. According to the chemiosmotic hypo-thesis, the coupling is effected through the generation of an electro-chemical proton gradient across the thylakoid membrane. This gradient then drives the synthesis of ATP through an ATPase acting in reverse (figure 4.3). It has been calculated that the pH inside thylakoids on illumination may be more than 2.5 units lower than that in the stroma; that is, the proton concentration inside is over 300 times that outside the thylakoids.

The dark reaction

Carbon-dioxide assimilation

In the second stage (dark reaction) of photosynthesis, carbon dioxide is assimilated into organic compounds in reactions which require the NADPH and ATP generated in the light reaction.

The chemical mechanisms involved in the uptake of carbon dioxide remained largely unknown until ^{14}C, the radioactive isotope of carbon, became available in the mid-1940s. Then Calvin and his associates carried out a series of experiments in which the incorporation of radioisotope from carbon dioxide into photosynthetic products was followed. They found that the green alga *Chlorella* when illuminated would take up the labelled carbon dioxide, and that within a few minutes a large number of compounds became labelled. By decreasing the time of exposure to $[^{14}C]$ carbon dioxide to about 2 seconds, Benson and Calvin were able to show that the first labelled product of photosynthesis was 3-phosphoglycerate. Other compounds only became labelled as the incubation time was increased.

These experiments showed that 3-phosphoglycerate was the primary product of photosynthetic carbon dioxide fixation. Over the next five years, a search was made for the acceptor of the carbon dioxide, which at that time was proposed to be a phosphorylated two-carbon compound.

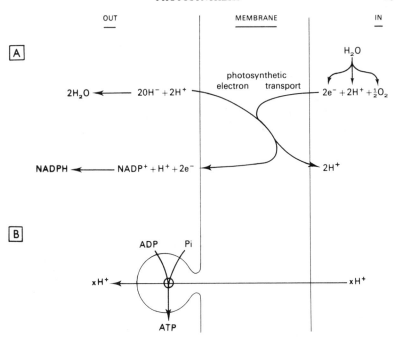

Figure 4.3 Photophosphorylation in thylakoids. According to the theory of Mitchell, the electron transport system is organized vectorially in the thylakoid membrane so that an electrochemical gradient is generated, with a high relative concentration of protons in the intrathylakoid space (A). This is then used to generate ATP by a coupling ATPase (B) plugged into the membrane.

Eventually Calvin and Wilson carried out the experiment illustrated in figure 4.4. Algae were allowed to carry out photosynthesis at a steady rate in the presence of excess (1%) carbon dioxide. The concentration of carbon dioxide was then decreased to a rate-limiting 0.003%, and the time course of changes in the concentrations of intermediates was followed. As expected, there was an immediate fall in the concentration of 3-phosphoglycerate as its rate of production through carbon dioxide fixation was decreased while its further metabolism continued unaltered (at least for a short time). More important was the fact that there was an immediate increase in the concentration of another compound, ribulose 1,5-bisphosphate. The time course of this increase was virtually a mirror image of the decrease in 3-phosphoglycerate. It was therefore suggested that ribulose 1,5-bisphosphate is the substrate for the carbon dioxide fixation reaction. Subsequent work has established that this is indeed the case.

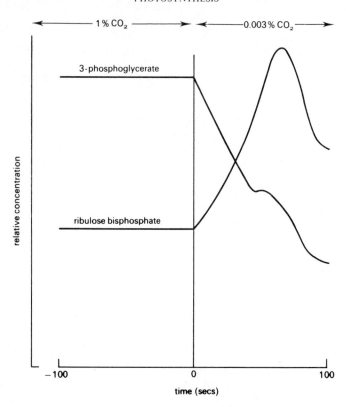

Figure 4.4 Effects of a sudden carbon-dioxide limitation on the concentrations of photosynthetic intermediates (redrawn from Calvin and Wilson, 1955).

The enzyme catalysing this reaction is ribulose bisphosphate carboxylase. Carboxylation of the substrate produces 2-carboxy-3-keto-ribitol 1,5-bisphosphate as intermediate, and this then gives two molecules of 3-phosphoglycerate:

$$
\begin{array}{c}
CH_2OP \\
| \\
C{=}O \\
| \\
HCOH \\
| \\
HCOH \\
| \\
CH_2OP
\end{array}
+ CO_2 \rightarrow
\left[
\begin{array}{c}
CH_2OP \\
| \\
{}^-OOC{-}COH \\
\text{------+------} \\
C{=}O \\
| \\
HCOH \\
| \\
CH_2OP
\end{array}
\right]
\rightarrow 2
\begin{array}{c}
COO^- \\
| \\
HCOH \\
| \\
CH_2OP
\end{array}
$$

The enzyme is present in large quantities in photosynthetic tissues, forming up to 50% of the total soluble leaf protein in some plants. The concentration of carbon dioxide in the atmosphere is rather low (0.03%), and the initial reaction of carbon assimilation is often rate-limiting under conditions of high light intensities. The large amounts of ribulose bisphosphate carboxylase found in chloroplasts can thus be seen as an adaptation to maximize carbon-dioxide fixation. In some plants there are additional mechanisms for ensuring that atmospheric carbon dioxide is absorbed efficiently for photosynthesis (p. 80).

Recycling of carbon

While carbon dioxide is being fixed in the ribulose bisphosphate carboxylase reaction, there is a requirement to provide the second substrate of the reaction—ribulose bisphosphate—at a rate equal to that of carbon-dioxide incorporation. This is achieved by a cyclic process known as the *Calvin cycle* in which 3-phosphoglycerate is converted to ribulose bisphosphate. Since the product of the ribulose bisphosphate carboxylase reaction contains 6 carbons (2 molecules of phosphoglycerate), whereas the substrate has 5 carbons, only 5/6 of the phosphoglycerate needs to be recycled back to ribulose bisphosphate to maintain substrate supply for the carboxylase. The remaining 1/6 (representing the carbon fixed from carbon dioxide) is in excess of the requirements of the cycle and can therefore be used for synthesis of cell materials which are the overall products of photosynthesis.

The reactions of the Calvin cycle are shown in figure 4.5. In many respects, the pathway resembles the pentose phosphate pathway of glucose metabolism (p. 52), and many of the reactions of the two pathways are identical. A difference between the pathways is that the overall flow of intermediates is in opposite directions: the oxidative pentose phosphate pathway brings about oxidation of substrate to carbon dioxide, whereas the Calvin cycle leads to reduction of substrate and uptake of carbon dioxide. Some additional reactions take place in the Calvin cycle. One of these is the conversion of 3-phosphoglycerate to glyceraldehyde 3-phosphate by the phosphoglycerate kinase and glyceraldehyde phosphate dehydrogenase reactions. In chloroplasts, the dehydrogenase is specific for NADPH (rather than the NADH of the glycolytic enzyme). The cycle also requires sedoheptulose 1,7-bisphosphatase and ribulose 5-phosphate kinase.

The stoichiometry of the Calvin cycle is such that, for every 3 molecules

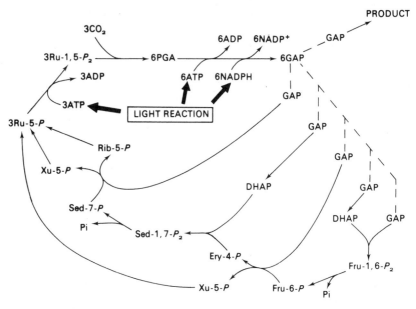

Figure 4.5 The Calvin cycle. Abbreviations are:

GAP	= glyceraldehyde 3-phosphate	DHAP = dihydroxyacetone phosphate
Ery-4-P	= erythrose 4-phosphate	PGA = 3-phosphoglycerate
Rib-5-P	= ribose 5-phosphate	Ru-5-P = ribulose 5-phosphate
Ru-1,5-P_2	= ribulose 1,5-bisphosphate	Sed-7-P = sedoheptulose 7-phosphate
Sed-1,7-P_2	= sedoheptulose 1,7-bisphosphate	Xu-5-P = xylulose 5-phosphate

of carbon dioxide fixed, one triose phosphate is produced, and a further 3 molecules of pentose are recycled back to ribulose bisphosphate. For each molecule of triose phosphate synthesized, there is also a requirement for 6 molecules of NADPH (for reduction of 6 molecules of phosphoglycerate at the glyceraldehyde phosphate dehydrogenase reaction) and 9 molecules of ATP (6 at glyceraldehyde phosphate dehydrogenase and 3 at ribulose 5-phosphate kinase). It is through these coenzyme requirements that the dark reactions of photosynthesis are coupled to the light reactions which generate the NADPH and ATP.

Products of photosynthesis

The immediate product of photosynthesis as represented in figure 4.5 is triose phosphate. This never accumulates in cells in significant quantities but is converted into other products, the nature of which can vary according to the species of plant.

One of the most common products is the polysaccharide starch, which accumulates in chloroplasts during daytime illumination and is then used during the night. In fact, this is the only major product to accumulate within the chloroplast. Most other products are synthesized in other parts of the cell, so that their precursors have to cross the chloroplast membrane.

The chloroplast inner membrane, like that of mitochondria, is selectively permeable to only certain substrates. Figure 4.6 shows a scheme for the transport of metabolites across the chloroplast membrane. An important role is played by the transport of dihydroxyacetone phosphate out of chloroplasts. This provides not only the carbon precursor, but also some of the ATP and reducing power required for many synthetic reactions. Chloroplasts are not permeable to NADPH or ATP, so these compounds can only be transported indirectly by means of a substrate cycle, similar in

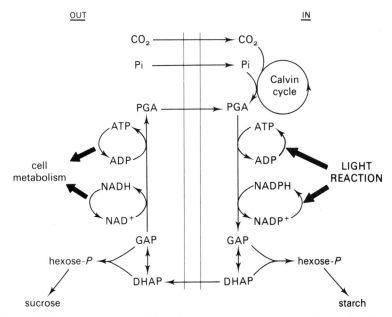

Figure 4.6 Transport across the chloroplast membrane during photosynthesis. The scheme shows two aspects of transport: (1) Carbon dioxide and orthophosphate are taken up by chloroplasts, and triose phosphate is exported to be used in synthetic reactions such as· sucrose synthesis. (2) Reducing equivalents and ATP generated by the light reaction are exported indirectly by a triose-phosphate shuttle system.

principle to those described for mitochondria (p. 35). In the dihydroxy-acetone phosphate/3-phosphoglycerate cycle shown in figure 4.6, phosphoglycerate is phosphorylated and reduced to triose phosphate at the expense of ATP and NADPH generated photosynthetically inside the chloroplast. Dihydroxyacetone phosphate can then pass out of the chloroplast and be converted back to phosphoglycerate by reactions linked to ATP synthesis and NAD^+ reduction. The cycle is completed by re-entry of the phosphoglycerate into the chloroplast.

A major product of photosynthesis in many plants is the disaccharide sucrose, which is used for transport of carbohydrate to other parts of the plant. Sucrose is formed in the cytosol from triose phosphates by gluconeogenesis (p. 62) and the UDP-glucose pathway (p. 99). The proportion of photosynthetic product converted to sucrose can depend on the age of the leaf. In immature leaves, much of the product is retained within the leaf for growth of more leaf tissue, and sucrose is only a minor product. In mature leaves, a large proportion of the product is trans-located as sucrose to other parts of the plant, where it can be stored or used for growth of other tissues. For this reason, the nature of the photosynthetic products can vary not only according to the species of plant but also according to the stage of the growth.

In addition to carbohydrates, plants require many other organic compounds for the synthesis of cell components, and the products of photosynthesis are diverted to a wide range of amino acids, nucleotides and lipids. Under some conditions up to 30% of fixed carbon dioxide is converted to amino acids.

Associated reactions

The reactions of the Calvin cycle are common to all plants and constitute the only known process for the assimilation of carbon dioxide into carbohydrate. However, in some plants, additional mechanisms exist for ensuring a supply of carbon dioxide essential for the ribulose bisphos-phate carboxylase reaction of the Calvin cycle.

One of the properties of ribulose bisphosphate carboxylase is its rather low affinity (high K_m) for carbon dioxide relative to the low concen-tration of carbon dioxide in the atmosphere. Some plants have evolved special mechanisms which are believed to increase the efficiency of carbon-dioxide uptake. These are the so-called "C-4 plants". In such plants, the first products labelled on exposure to $[^{14}C]$ carbon dioxide are a group of 4-carbon compounds—oxaloacetate, malate and aspartate—

rather than the 3-phosphoglycerate found in the more usual "C-3 plants".

Sugar cane and maize are examples of such C-4 plants. The leaves contain two different cell types involved in photosynthesis. The inner "bundle sheath" cells contain ribulose bisphosphate carboxylase as their main carbon-dioxide fixing system, whereas the outer "mesophyll" cells contain phosphoenolpyruvate carboxylase. Carbon dioxide fixation in these plants is proposed to involve cooperation between these two cell types. Carbon dioxide is first fixed in the mesophyll cells by the phosphoenolpyruvate carboxylase reaction to give oxaloacetate. The oxaloacetate is reduced to malate and transported to the bundle sheath cells, where carbon dioxide is released by oxidative decarboxylation of the malate. The carbon dioxide is then fixed by the ribulose bisphosphate carboxylase, and the other product of malate decarboxylation (pyruvate) is returned to the mesophyll cells. The cycle is completed by phosphorylation of pyruvate to phosphoenolpyruvate by pyruvate, orthophosphate dikinase (p. 64).

Variations of this scheme have been found in other plant species. Thus, in some plants, aspartate is transported from mesophyll to bundle sheath layer and, after decarboxylation, alanine is returned to the mesophyll layer. However, the basic features of carbon dioxide metabolism in all C-4 plants seem to be the same: carbon dioxide fixation in the outer layer of cells, transport of a C-4 product to the inner cells where the carbon dioxide is released for photosynthetic assimilation, and return of C-3 product to the outer layer.

This scheme, therefore, operates as a "pump" to concentrate carbon dioxide in the inner bundle sheath cells. The advantage is that phosphoenolpyruvate carboxylase has a high affinity for CO_2 and is a more effective scavenger of carbon dioxide than ribulose bisphosphate carboxylase. Thus atmospheric carbon dioxide can be taken up more efficiently, and across a greater concentration gradient, than for C-3 plants which rely solely on ribulose bisphosphate carboxylase. This has two physiological advantages. Firstly, the plants can make more effective use of high light intensities at which carbon dioxide uptake would otherwise become a limiting factor. Secondly, because the uptake mechanism for carbon dioxide is more efficient, the stomata (pores) on the leaf surface do not need to allow as rapid an exchange of air between the internal airspace of the leaf and the outside atmosphere. This means that water loss through transpiration (which inevitably accompanies air exchange) is less than is possible in C-3 plants. Typically, C-4 plants live in tropical climates where the high light intensity and limited water availability give a selective advantage to this type of plant. Under these conditions, they synthesize about twice as much organic material as C-3 plants.

A rather different system for maintaining carbon dioxide supplies for photosynthesis is found in plants of the family Crassulaceae and a few other families. Such plants are usually succulent and tend to live in arid regions. Here the leaf stomata are open during the night to allow air exchange. Carbon dioxide is then fixed by phosphoenolpyruvate carboxylase to give malate, phosphoenolpyruvate being supplied for this purpose by breakdown of starch reserves in the leaf. During daylight, the stomata close and carbon dioxide is released from malate to be used for photosynthesis by the ribulose bisphosphate carboxylase reaction and Calvin cycle. Since water loss by air exchange at night is less than it would be during the higher daytime temperatures, this process can be seen as another adaptation to restrict water loss from the leaves.

Photorespiration

Most plants, when illuminated, not only fix carbon dioxide by photosynthesis but also oxidize organic compounds to carbon dioxide in the specifically light-induced process of photorespiration. The relative rates of these two opposing reactions depend on the concentrations of carbon dioxide and oxygen in the atmosphere. With high carbon dioxide concentrations, photorespiration is suppressed so that photosynthesis is the dominant pathway. With low carbon dioxide concentrations and high oxygen concentrations, the rate of photorespiration increases to equal or even exceed that of photosynthesis.

An important reaction in photorespiration seems to be one in which ribulose bisphosphate reacts with oxygen to give 3-phosphoglycerate plus phosphoglycolate:

$$
\begin{array}{ccc}
CH_2OP & & CH_2OP \\
| & & | \\
C{=}O & & COO^- \\
| & & + \\
HCOH & +O_2 \rightarrow & COO^- \quad +2H^+ \\
| & & | \\
HCOH & & HCOH \\
| & & | \\
CH_2OP & & CH_2OP
\end{array}
$$

This is probably catalysed by ribulose bisphosphate çarboxylase in an alternative reaction to the normal one of carboxylation. According to this, the fate of ribulose bisphosphate (carboxylation or oxidation) depends on the relative concentrations of carbon dioxide and oxygen available to the enzyme. The further metabolism of phosphoglycolate proceeds by de-phosphorylation, oxidation to glyoxylate, and then conversion to glycine, serine, carbon dioxide and other products.

The function of photorespiration is not known for certain. One proposal is that it is a protective mechanism which allows the photo-systems to continue to turn over under conditions of bright illumination where carbon dioxide supply is rate-limiting for photosynthesis.

Photosynthetic microorganisms

A significant proportion (perhaps up to a half) of the total atmospheric carbon dioxide fixed by photosynthesis is carried out by microorganisms. There are several different photosynthetic types within the micro-organisms. A major division is between the eukaryotes, such as the green algae which have chloroplasts, and the prokaryotes which have no chloroplasts and are themselves considered to be equivalent in some ways to chloroplasts. All the eukaryotes studied seem to have essentially the same system as that already described for higher plants. Thus the unicellular green alga *Chlorella* was used by Calvin's group for their classical studies on photosynthesis. Such organisms have chloroplasts with two photosystems; they fix carbon dioxide, use water as electron donor, and produce molecular oxygen.

The photosynthetic prokaryotes include the blue-green algae or Cyanophyta (a completely different group from the eukaryotic green algae) and the photosynthetic bacteria. The blue-green algae have two photosystems and are able to use water as electron donor, but bacteria are unable to do this and, instead, use a variety of other electron donors, both inorganic and organic.

There are three main groups of photosynthetic bacteria. The green sulphur bacteria are strict anaerobes which use hydrogen sulphide as electron donor and oxidize it to sulphur. Some can further oxidize the sulphur to thiosulphate and sulphate, whereas others can use hydrogen gas as electron donor. The purple sulphur bacteria also oxidize hydrogen sulphide to sulphur, but have a rather different pigment system to that of the green sulphur bacteria. The third group is the non-sulphur bacteria, and these use organic compounds as electron donors; for example, isopropanol, pyruvate or ethanol are oxidized by organisms from this group. In some cases, an organic compound is also used as carbon source in place of carbon dioxide.

In prokaryotes, the light reactions of photosynthesis take place on membranes within the cell. In some, there is simply a pigmented region of the plasma membrane, whereas in others there are pigmented infoldings of the membrane specialized for photosynthesis and more resembling the thylakoids of plants. These can be isolated from some bacteria as "chromatophores" which can be used experimentally to study the light reactions of photosynthesis.

The actual light reaction in bacteria is simpler than that in plants in that only one photosystem is involved. This is because the electron donors used have much less positive redox potentials than that of water, so that the energy boost from one photosystem is enough to reduce a carrier of sufficiently negative potential to be able to reduce $NADP^+$.

Where carbon dioxide is used as carbon source, it is assimilated by the Calvin cycle. Bacteria are also able to use light-generated reducing power to reduce nitrate to ammonia (as in plants), and some are able to reduce nitrogen to ammonia. Such nitrogen-fixing photosynthetic bacteria are able to derive all of their carbon, hydrogen and oxygen from the air.

CHAPTER FIVE

TRANSPORT

Transport across membranes

The cytoplasm of all cells is separated from the external environment by the plasma membrane (plasmalemma). In common with other biological membranes, the plasma membrane has a lipid bilayer structure which is almost impermeable to most water-soluble organic molecules and to ions. This permeability barrier allows the cell to maintain an internal environment different from that of the external medium, and partially independent of it. The membrane is important in controlling the composition of solutes within the cell, so that metabolic reactions can take place under optimum conditions.

However, the membrane must allow some materials to pass through. Nutrients such as sugars and amino acids must be taken into cells, and excretory products must pass out of them. For all but the simplest molecules, simple diffusion does not contribute significantly to transport. Instead, there are components in the plasma membrane which specifically allow certain molecules or ions to pass through. These components are variously known as *transport systems, carriers, translocases, permeases* or *porters*, and the process by which they transport substrates is known as *facilitated diffusion* or *mediated transport.*

There is good evidence that these transport systems are specific proteins in the membrane. The properties of the transport systems resemble enzymes in a number of respects:

(1) They show saturation with substrate (i.e. Michaelis-Menten type of kinetics, rather than an unlimited concentration-dependent increase in transport rate as would be the case for simple diffusion).
(2) They show considerable specificity, and can distinguish between stereoisomers such as D-glucose and L-glucose.

(3) They may be inhibited by specific inhibitors.
(4) They may be inactivated by specific protein-reacting reagents.
(5) Iñ bacteria, at least, they are inherited genetically in a similar way to enzymes. Some are constitutive to bacteria, whereas others are induced only when suitable substrates are present in the external medium.

The detailed molecular mechanism by which the transport systems move substrates across membranes is not yet known. Because of their enzyme-like properties, it is believed that there must be a specific binding site on the protein rather similar to that of an enzyme active site. (Some bacterial surface proteins have been isolated and found to bind the appropriate substrates with similar kinetic properties and specificity characteristics to those of the transport systems.) However, it is not yet known how the transporter actually assists the substrate to cross the lipid membrane. In some older models, the carrier binds to substrate and then crosses the membrane or rotates within it before releasing the substrate at the opposite side. In more recent models, the transport protein extends across the membrane and has a hydrophilic pore to allow the substrate through. The pore contains a specific binding site for the substrate, and the protein may undergo a conformational change when it binds the substrate so that the substrate can pass through.

General types of membrane transport

There are three main types of membrane transport: *passive transport*, *active transport* and *group translocation*. These are shown diagrammatically in figure 5.1.

Passive transport into cells can occur only when the concentration of solute in the external medium is greater than the concentration in the cell. The direction of transport is always down a concentration gradient, so it is sometimes known as "downhill" transport. Because the process involves the dilution of solute (an exergonic reaction), there is no additional energy requirement for passive transport.

Active transport involves the "uphill" transport of substrate against a concentration gradient. Because this is an endergonic process, active transport requires some form of energy supply. Some active transport systems may use ATP directly as an energy source, but a more usual process is one in which the uphill transport of a substrate is coupled to the (exergonic) downhill transport of a secondary substrate or ion. Provided that the ratio of concentrations ("concentration gradient") of the primary substrate across the two sides of the membrane is less than the concentration gradient of the secondary component, the overall transport will be exergonic and proceed in the direction of uphill transport of the primary substrate. Bacteria frequently make use of a proton gradient to drive active transport reactions (p. 91), whereas in mammalian intestine a sodium ion gradient is used for the same purpose. Both of these systems involve the co-transport of the two solutes in the same direction ("symport"), but there is no reason why countertransport ("antiport") of the two solutes in opposite directions should not function equally well, provided that the appropriate concentration gradients exist. Some active transport processes are extremely effective in concentrating solutes, and concentration gradients of better than 1000 to 1 can be achieved. This is clearly of considerable advantage to bacteria growing in a medium containing only a low concentration of nutrients.

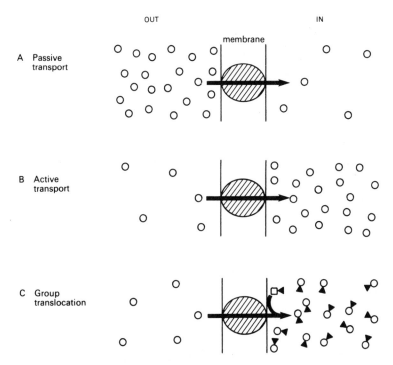

Figure 5.1   General mechanisms for membrane transport. In passive transport (A), molecules move from a compartment of high concentration to one of low concentration. In active transport (B), molecules move "uphill" to a compartment of higher concentration, and an external source of energy is required. In group translocation (C), the substrate is concentrated as a derivative which is not able to pass back through the membrane.

In the third type of transport system known as *group translocation* (figure 5.1C), the substrate is not only transported but is converted to a chemically different product during the transport process. Since the product may be accumulated within the cells at a higher concentration than that of the substrate outside, there is effectively an uphill transport of the substrate. Chemical energy is used to convert the substrate to its product. Group translocation is used by some bacteria to accumulate sugars, and the product of this reaction is sugar phosphate (p. 92).

Passive transport in animal cells

Blood glucose is available to mammalian tissues in relatively high concentrations, so that passive diffusion can be an effective process for transport into the cells. The properties of the transport system for glucose have been studied in a number of different tissues, and seem to be very similar if not identical in all of them. Thus the transport systems of erythrocytes, skeletal muscle, heart and adipose tissue show the same substrate specificity and can transport D-glucose, D-mannose, D-galactose, 3-O-methyl glucose and 2-deoxy glucose by the same carrier. D-Fructose is not transported by the same system, however.

Despite having identical or near-identical transport systems, different tissues may respond in different ways to hormonal regulation of sugar transport. Insulin stimulates the uptake of glucose by such tissues as muscle and adipose tissue which have the receptors to respond to this hormone. However, in red blood cells and liver, insulin has little or no effect on glucose transport, even though other processes in liver are insulin-sensitive (p. 178).

In skeletal muscle, the transport of glucose is stimulated during muscle contraction and under conditions of low oxygen tension. Under both of these physiological conditions, the muscle requires an increased substrate supply because of the increased requirements for energy production by glycolysis. On the other hand, when alternative substrates such as fatty acids are available, there may be a decrease in the rate of glucose uptake.

Active transport in animal cells

The two main sites of active transport of sugars in mammalian tissues are the small intestine and the kidney. In the intestine, the concentration of glucose in the lumen (digestive region) may vary considerably (depending on whether a carbohydrate-containing meal is being digested or not) but will often be much lower than that of the blood. Hence the need for active transport of glucose from the lumen to the blood. In the kidney, excretion involves filtration of the blood, followed by reabsorption of glucose and other useful components. Active transport is required to maintain the glucose concentration in the urine at a much lower level than that of blood.

The active transport systems of intestine and kidney are similar to each other, but differ from the passive transport systems of other tissues. Not only does the active system have the ability to carry out uphill transport, but it has a different substrate specificity from the passive system. Thus, although D-glucose and D-galactose are transported by both systems, D-mannose is not a substrate for the active system. The active system also has a requirement for sodium ions not shown by the passive system, and indeed this is essential to provide the driving force for uphill transport (see below).

The epithelial cells of the small intestine and kidney tubule cells are both rather unusual in having two different sides, with the membranes of the two sides having different properties. For the intestinal cell, it is the luminal or brush border membrane (the digestive side) which has the active transport system for sugars (figure 5.2). The contraluminal membrane which is in contact with the blood capillaries has different morphological and biochemical properties from the luminal membrane. The

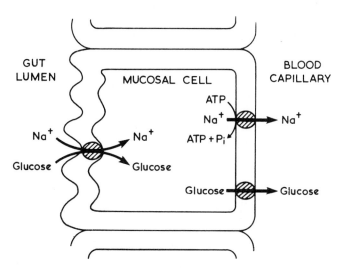

Figure 5.2 Transport of glucose across the mammalian intestine.

contraluminal membrane possesses an active transport system for pumping sodium ions out of the cell, and the energy for this process is provided by ATP hydrolysis. The sodium pump maintains the sodium ions within the cell at a low concentration, so that a gradient exists between this and the higher concentration of sodium ions in the lumen. This gradient provides the driving force for sugar transport. There is obligatory coupling between the entry of a sugar molecule and that of a sodium ion, and neither can enter the cell alone. A 1:1 stoichiometric relationship exists between entry of sugar and entry of sodium ions. The favourable concentration gradient of sodium ions for entry into the cell is used to move glucose against a concentration gradient. In addition to the concentration gradient, there is also a transmembrane potential with the interior of the cell at a negative potential relative to the outside. This reinforces the tendency of sodium ions to enter the cell. In this way, the sodium pump at the contraluminal plasma membrane indirectly provides the driving force for active transport of glucose at the luminal membrane. The active transport system maintains a higher concentration of glucose within the mucosal cells than that of the blood plasma. The glucose can then pass from the cells into the blood by a passive transport system present in the contraluminal membrane.

A similar arrangement exists in the kidney tubule cell. Active transport on a sodium ion gradient carries glucose from the tubule into the cells. The sugar is then released into the blood through the passive transport system at the opposite face of the cell.

The active transport of glucose by the intestine is partly responsible for maintaining a high concentration of glucose in blood. Fructose, on the other hand, is not an important blood sugar. It appears in the blood only transiently after fructose or sucrose has been ingested, and is rapidly metabolized by the liver and other tissues. The concentration gradient between intestine and blood is therefore nearly always favourable for fructose absorption. In keeping with this, it is found that fructose is absorbed through a facilitated transport system.

Active transport in bacteria

Unlike animal systems where many tissues use passive transport, most of the systems in bacteria involve active accumulation of substrates. The active transport of sugars in microorganisms may be of two general types. In the first type, the uphill transport of substrate may be coupled to the downhill transport of a secondary substance, according to the principle established for sugar transport on a sodium gradient in mammalian intestine. In bacteria, a proton gradient frequently provides the driving force for such active transport. In the second type, the energy for active transport may come more directly from ATP hydrolysis.

The ability to maintain a proton gradient across the membrane is found in bacteria, mitochondria and chloroplasts. According to the theories first proposed by P. Mitchell, oxidation of substrates by the respiratory chain is coupled to the ejection of protons from the cell or organelle, so that the exergonic reactions of substrate oxidation are used to form an electro-chemical gradient. This consists of a concentration gradient of protons, combined with a transmembrane potential with the interior negative. The potential for protons to return is a combination of both of these factors and is referred to as the proton motive force (p.m.f.). Once formed, this gradient can be made to do work of various types, including ATP synthesis and the concentration of substrates against an adverse gradient. The transport of lactose into *Escherichia coli* is an extensively studied example of this process of active transport (figure 5.3).

The second type of active transport system is found in Gram-negative bacteria and involves ATP hydrolysis. Such systems have substrate binding proteins which may be located in the periplasmic space outside the plasma membrane but inside the outer membrane (p. 131). In some

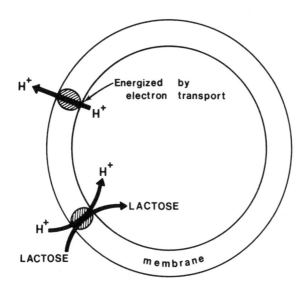

Figure 5.3 Proton-dependent active transport of lactose in bacteria.

bacteria, these proteins can be experimentally released into the medium by osmotic shock, and are found to have the same kinetic and specificity properties as the transport systems of the bacteria. The binding proteins generally have a high affinity for their substrates, and are therefore very effective in scavenging nutrients from dilute solutions. It has been proposed that once the substrate is inside the cell, the affinity between substrate and protein is decreased by an energy-dependent process which is directly or indirectly linked to ATP hydrolysis.

Group translocation in bacteria

Group translocation involves the conversion of sugars to sugar phosphates during the process of transport into the cell. The phosphate group is derived from phosphoenolpyruvate, but the phosphorylation is not direct and takes place via a series of protein carriers (figure 5.4). This system for sugar transport is known as the phosphotransferase or PTS system. Some components of the system (those on the right-hand side in the figure) are common to the transport of many sugars, whereas the components on the left (Enzyme II complex and Enzyme III) are more sugar-specific. To transport several different sugars, the bacterium may require a corresponding number of different sugar-specific components, all operating through the same general components. The sugar-specific components are associated with the membrane, but the other components are intracellular.

The PTS system for sugar transport is found mainly in bacteria which can grow under anaerobic conditions. The product of transport can be used directly for glycolysis, so that the hexokinase reaction is bypassed in such bacteria.

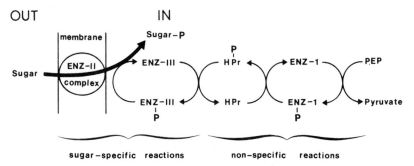

Figure 5.4   PTS group translocation in bacteria.

Transport in extracellular fluids

The transport of carbohydrates between different tissues in multi-cellular organisms takes place by means of specific transport sugars. In vertebrates, glucose is the transport form of carbohydrate in the blood, and other sugars are rarely accumulated in the blood in significant quantities. Various homeostatic mechanisms have evolved to maintain the concentration of glucose in blood to within a narrow concentration range (around 5 mM for many mammals). The liver is important in this homeostasis, taking up excess glucose after digestion of a meal and releasing it again later. In addition, many other tissues respond to hormonal stimulation (e.g. by insulin) by altering their rate of glucose uptake and metabolism (p. 182).

Insects and some other invertebrates have the disaccharide trehalose as their main blood sugar. It occurs in much higher concentrations than glucose in mammalian blood and may have some advantages as a transport sugar (p. 98).

Most higher plants employ sucrose to transport carbohydrate between different tissues, and this also has advantages (p. 100). Sucrose is transported from photosynthesizing leaves to other tissues (shoots, roots, storage tissues) in the phloem. Since the concentration of sugar in the phloem may be higher than in the leaves, active transport is required to load the sugars into the sieve tubes which carry the phloem. The detailed properties of such transport systems are less clearly known than for microbial and mammalian systems, but there is some evidence that a proton gradient may be required to drive the reaction. In germinating seeds and sprouting storage organs, the stored polysaccharides are also converted to sucrose for transport to the growing tissues.

Other transport carbohydrates in plants include oligosaccharides such as raffinose (p. 101) and the sugar alcohols D-glucitol, D-mannitol, and D-galactitol (p. 46). It may be significant that all of these compounds, like sucrose and trehalose, are non-reducing carbohydrates.

CHAPTER SIX

GLYCOSIDES AND OLIGOSACCHARIDES

Glycosides are compounds in which two components are linked together. The first component is the glycosyl group which is derived from a reducing sugar in which the anomeric hydroxyl group has been substituted. The second component can either be a second carbohydrate, as in oligosaccharides and polysaccharides, or can be some other compound or "aglycone" such as an alcohol, a phenol, an amide or an amine.

The most common types of glycosides are the O-glycosides in which an oxygen atom links the two components. However, N-glycosides and S-glycosides also occur, in which nitrogen or sulphur atoms link the two parts of the molecule (figure 6.1).

Biosynthesis of glycosides

The enzymic synthesis of glycosides occurs through transfer reactions in which a sugar linked through its anomeric carbon to a donor group is transferred to a suitable acceptor molecule. The donor group is most commonly a nucleoside diphosphate, but transfer reactions can also occur from groups such as phosphate, other sugars or inositol. The general equation for such reactions is:

$$\text{sugar-donor} + \text{acceptor} \rightleftharpoons \text{donor} + \text{sugar-acceptor}$$

The equilibrium position of such transfer reactions depends upon the relative free energies of hydrolysis of the sugar-donor and the sugar-acceptor. If the sugar-donor has a higher free energy of hydrolysis than the sugar-acceptor, then the transfer reaction equilibrium will be in favour of sugar-acceptor formation. Such is the case when a nucleoside diphosphate sugar is the glycosyl donor—the free energy of hydrolysis of the glycosyl-phosphate bond of such compounds is higher than that of most glycosides. This drives the transfer reactions in the direction of glycoside synthesis, and is probably one of the main reasons for the wide use of nucleoside diphosphate sugars as glycoside precursors in many biological systems.

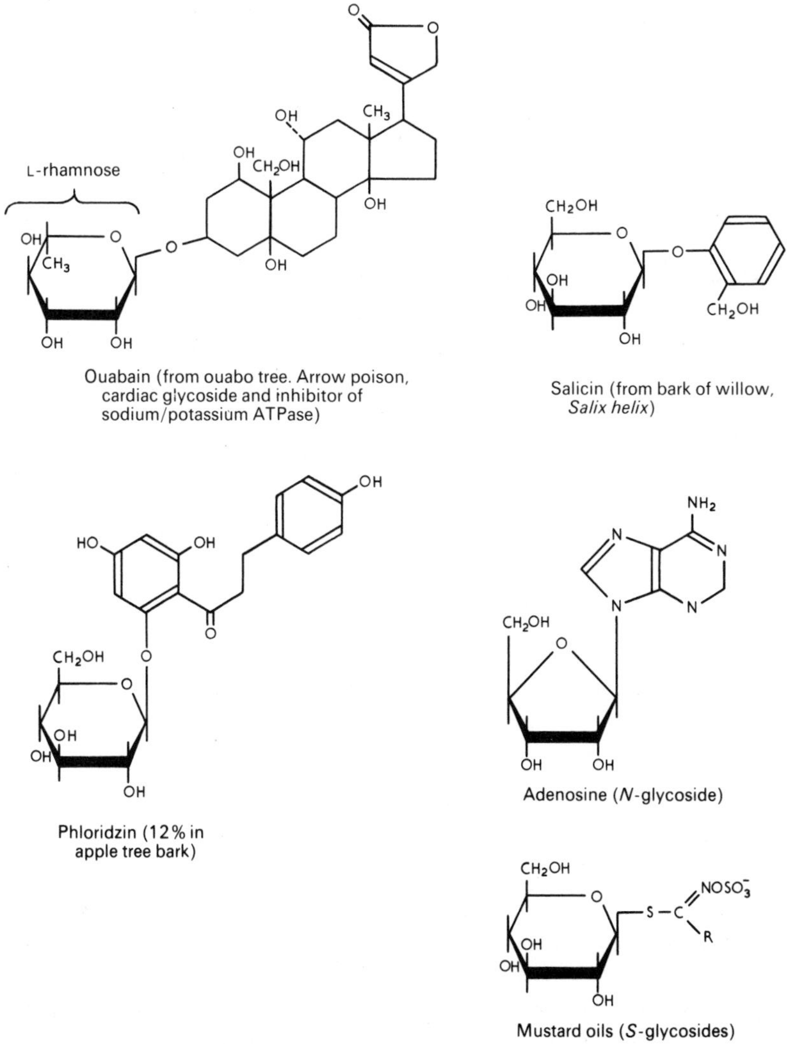

Ouabain (from ouabo tree. Arrow poison, cardiac glycoside and inhibitor of sodium/potassium ATPase)

Salicin (from bark of willow, *Salix helix*)

Phloridzin (12% in apple tree bark)

Adenosine (*N*-glycoside)

Mustard oils (*S*-glycosides)

Figure 6.1 Structures of some naturally-occurring glycosides.

Less commonly, glycosides are formed in reactions not directly involving nucleoside diphosphate sugars. One example is in the synthesis of extracellular polysaccharides in some microorganisms. Nucleotides do not normally pass through plasma membranes, so that internally-generated nucleoside diphosphate sugars cannot be used for synthesis of polysaccharides outside the membrane. Bacteria (*Streptococcus mutans*) which colonize teeth and are responsible for the formation of dental caries, make use of sucrose as a precursor for the synthesis of glucan (a polysaccharide of glucose).

$$\text{sucrose} + (\text{glucose})_n \overset{\text{dextransucrase}}{\rightleftharpoons} \text{fructose} + (\text{glucose})_{n+1}$$

The free energy of hydrolysis of the glycosidic bond in sucrose is higher than that of the glucan, so polysaccharide formation is favoured.

Plants also make use of transglycosylation reactions from sucrose for the synthesis of inulin (p. 128), and use galactosyl-inositol as the precursor of galactosyl residues in raffinose and related oligosaccharides (p. 101).

Whatever the immediate precursor of the glycoside, free sugars are nearly always converted to phosphate derivatives before further metabolism can take place. A typical reaction sequence in the synthesis of a glucoside from free glucose is:

(1) $\text{ATP} + \text{glucose} \overset{\text{hexokinase}}{\longrightarrow} \text{glucose 6-phosphate} + \text{ADP}$

(2) $\text{glucose 6-phosphate} \overset{\text{phosphoglucomutase}}{\rightleftharpoons} \text{glucose 1-phosphate}$

(3) $\text{glucose 1-phosphate} + \text{UTP} \overset{\substack{\text{glucose-1-phosphate} \\ \text{uridylyl transferase}}}{\rightleftharpoons} \text{UDP-glucose} + \text{pyrophosphate}$

$$\downarrow \text{pyrophosphatase}$$
$$2\,\text{P}_i$$

(4) $\text{UDP-glucose} + \text{acceptor} \overset{\text{glucosyltransferase}}{\longrightarrow} \text{glucosyl-acceptor} + \text{UDP}$

Note that glucose 6-phosphate is first converted to glucose 1-phosphate before nucleoside diphosphate sugar formation. This is because nucleoside diphosphate sugars always have the sugars linked through the glycosidic carbon (C-1 for glucose). In many tissues nucleoside diphosphate sugar formation is favoured because of the presence of a pyrophosphatase which removes the second product of the uridylyl transferase reaction.

Disaccharides

The two most widely-occurring disaccharides in biology are sucrose and trehalose, both of which are important in the transport and storage of carbohydrate. In addition, lactose has a more restricted distribution, but has also received considerable attention as the main carbohydrate of milk, and therefore of the diet of newborn mammals. These three disaccharides are all synthesized specifically to perform essential functions. Many other disaccharides also occur biologically, but arise as products of the partial hydrolysis of polysaccharides and are not usually specifically synthesized as such. For example, maltose appears during the hydrolysis of starch and glycogen (p. 114) but is only a transient intermediate and appears to have no other biological function. Oligosaccharides which usually appear only during the hydrolysis of polymers will not be considered further in this chapter.

Trehalose

In trehalose, two D-glucose residues are joined together through their glycosidic carbons to give a non-reducing disaccharide in which both monosaccharide residues are identical (figure 6.2). In naturally-occurring trehalose, the glycosidic link is α with respect to both glucosyl residues.

Trehalose has been found in insects and a wide variety of other invertebrates, actinomycetes, fungi, yeasts and some higher plants. The mechanism for synthesis of trehalose appears to be the same in animals and plants. Two enzymes are involved—trehalose phosphate synthase and trehalose phosphatase:

$$UDP\text{-}Glc + Glc\text{-}6\text{-}P \rightarrow Trehalose\text{-}6\text{-}P + UDP$$
$$Trehalose\text{-}6\text{-}P \rightarrow Trehalose + Pi$$

This two-stage reaction for trehalose synthesis may have an advantage over a more direct mechanism (transfer to free glucose rather than glucose 6-phosphate as acceptor) in that the equilibrium of the second reaction is strongly in favour of trehalose formation. This ensures that trehalose

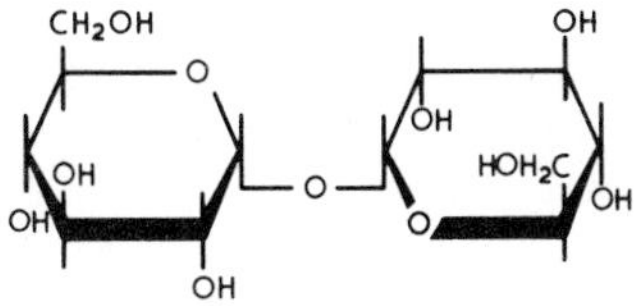

Figure 6.2   Trehalose (α-D-glucopyranosyl-α-D-glucopyranoside).

synthesis proceeds to completion and is physiologically irreversible, so that high concentrations of trehalose can be formed under conditions where concentrations of precursors are relatively low.

Trehalose synthesis is favoured under conditions where there is an ample carbohydrate supply—in yeast grown with excess glucose or in fed insects. It is then used later during times of carbohydrate requirement, such as during starvation in yeast or during flight or metamorphosis in insects. In addition to this storage function, trehalose has a transport function in some organisms. In insects, carbohydrate is stored in the fat body as glycogen which can be converted to trehalose for transport in the blood to other tissues such as muscle. In most insects, and in some other invertebrates, trehalose is the main blood sugar rather than glucose, and it may reach concentrations of 2% or more, some twenty times the concentration of glucose in mammalian blood.

A number of suggestions have been made as to why trehalose rather than glucose is used for transport and storage of carbohydrate. Its wide distribution in invertebrates and lower plants suggests that it must have evolutionary advantages. One may be that twice as much carbohydrate can be stored as trehalose than as glucose for the same contribution to osmotic pressure, and yet trehalose is sufficiently soluble to be freely transported in solution. Another advantage may lie in the relative chemical inertness of trehalose, a non-reducing sugar. A role in insects may be related to the transport of monosaccharides from the gut lumen in the blood. The gut epithelia of insects (unlike mammals, p. 89) apparently do not possess an active mechanism for monosaccharide transport. Instead, monosaccharides pass reversibly across the epithelium by facilitated diffusion. Rapid conversion of monosaccharides to trehalose by the fat body (which lies immediately around the gut) acts as an effective trap, because the disaccharide is unable to diffuse across the gut wall.

The main mechanism by which trehalose is metabolized is through hydrolysis to glucose in a reaction catalysed by trehalase. One exception to the hydrolytic mechanism of trehalose utilization is known: *Euglena gracilis* possesses a trehalose phosphorylase which catalyses the phosphorolytic breakdown of trehalose to glucose plus glucose 1-phosphate:

$$\text{trehalose} + \text{Pi} \rightleftharpoons \text{glucose} + \text{glucose-1-}P$$

Sucrose

Like trehalose, sucrose is a non-reducing disaccharide. It consists of an α-glucopyranose residue linked to a β-fructofuranose residue (figure 1.11).

Most photosynthetic plants produce sucrose as the main soluble product of photosynthesis, and it is as sucrose that carbohydrate is transported from photosynthetic tissues to other parts of the plant. The mechanism of synthesis is similar to that of trehalose in that a disaccharide-phosphate is an intermediate:

$$\text{UDP-Glc} + \text{Fru-6-}P \overset{\text{sucrose phosphate synthase}}{\rightleftharpoons} \text{UDP} + \text{sucrose-6-}P$$

$$\text{sucrose-6-}P \overset{\text{sucrose-6-phosphatase}}{\longrightarrow} \text{sucrose} + \text{Pi}$$

The equilibrium of the overall process is very much in favour of sucrose synthesis, so high concentrations of sucrose can be produced from low concentrations of precursors. Some plants also contain an enzyme which catalyses transfer of glucose from UDP-glucose onto free fructose:

$$\text{UDP-Glc} + \text{Fru} \overset{\text{sucrose synthase}}{\rightleftharpoons} \text{sucrose} + \text{UDP}$$

However, because the free energy of hydrolysis of the glycosidic link of sucrose is unusually high (see below), the equilibrium is not strongly in favour of sucrose synthesis. At the concentration of metabolites in the cell, the enzyme may catalyse the reverse reaction, leading to sucrose break-down and formation of UDP-glucose.

The biological functions of sucrose are similar to those of trehalose—it serves both to transport and store carbohydrate. The transport function is important in nearly all higher plants, but the storage function varies considerably according to the species. Man has made particular use of the sugar cane, where in cultivated varieties, the concentration of stored sucrose in the stem can be as high as 16%. Sugar beet also has a high sucrose content, and these two plants are the main sources from which table sugar is made.

The metabolic fate of sucrose is more varied than that of trehalose, as sucrose is frequently used for synthesis of polysaccharides in storage tissues. It is known to be metabolized by at least three different types of reaction. The first is hydrolysis to the component monosaccharides:

$$\text{sucrose} + H_2O \rightarrow \text{fructose} + \text{glucose}$$

The trivial name of "invertase" for enzymes which catalyse this hydrolysis arises from the observation that dextrorotatory sucrose is converted to a laevorotary mixture of monosaccharides. There is thus an "inversion" of rotation which can be followed in a polarimeter. Enzymes which hydrolyse sucrose can be either α-glucosidases or β-fructosidases.

Sucrose can also be degraded by sucrose synthase. As noted above, this reaction has an equilibrium position close to unity, unlike the equivalent reactions for synthesis of most other glycosides. If the product (UDP-Glc) of this reaction is removed by further metabolism, such as polysaccharide formation, then the reaction will proceed in the direction of sucrose breakdown. High concentrations of sucrose also favour UDP-glucose formation.

The third group of reactions for metabolism of sucrose are trans-glycosylations in which polysaccharides such as glucan (p. 96) and inulin (p. 128) can be formed directly. Again, because of the large free energy of hydrolysis of sucrose relative to most other glycosides, such reactions favour synthesis of the other glycosides at the expense of sucrose.

Some of the advantages of sucrose as a transport sugar are similar to those of trehalose. It is a disaccharide with half the osmotic effect of an equivalent weight of monosaccharide, and it is chemically less reactive than its component monosaccharides. Sucrose may have additional advantages of its own to the plant. Its unusually high free energy of hydrolysis gives it the potential to be metabolized in the several different ways described above. This high free energy of hydrolysis is partly due to the presence of the β-fructofuranose residue in the molecule. Thus the equilibrium of hydrolysis may be particularly favoured by partial removal of one of the immediate products of the reaction, β-fructofuranose, by its isomerization to the rather lower-energy pyranose forms:

$$\text{sucrose} \rightarrow \alpha\text{-glucopyranose} + \beta\text{-fructofuranose}$$
$$\Updownarrow \qquad\qquad \Updownarrow$$
$$\beta\text{-glucopyranose} \quad \alpha\text{-fructofuranose,}$$
$$\alpha\text{-fructopyranose,}$$
$$\beta\text{-fructopyranose}$$

Sucrose is one of the sweetest-tasting sugars and has become an important part of the human diet in many countries. The daily intake in Britain averages over 100 grams per person, representing about 20% of the total calorie intake. This high sucrose diet has only developed over the past hundred years or so, since the manufacture of refined sugar became widespread. A number of diseases of modern man have been ascribed to this high intake of sucrose. For example, there is little doubt that formation of dental caries is promoted by sucrose-containing foods. There is also evidence that the incidence of diabetes is increased in human populations which have a high intake of dietary sucrose.

Rather more controversial is the possible effect of sucrose-containing diets on the incidence of coronary thrombosis and related diseases of the blood vessels and heart. Several comparative studies of human populations show a positive correlation between the average sucrose intake in the diet and frequency of this type of disease. However, because it is difficult to rule out other differences between the compared populations, the effect of sucrose on coronary thrombosis is not firmly established. One problem in studying this effect is that several factors can contribute to the incidence of heart disease, and it is difficult to isolate a single factor such as the content of sucrose in the diet. Thus populations which have a high sucrose intake tend to be the more affluent populations and, associated with this, is a tendency to overeat, to take less exercise, and to smoke more—factors which may also be linked with heart disease.

Plant oligosaccharides

In addition to sucrose, a number of plants synthesize oligosaccharides containing three or more monosaccharide residues. These have similar functions to sucrose in transport and storage of carbohydrate.

The most common group of such oligosaccharides is the raffinose family. These are derivatives of sucrose in which the glucosyl residue of the disaccharide is further substituted with one or more galactose residues to give raffinose (a trisaccharide), stachyose (tetrasaccharide), and verbascose (pentasaccharide) (figure 6.3). These oligosaccharides are synthesized from sucrose by an unusual transfer reaction in which a galactoside of inositol, known as galactinol, is the immediate galactosyl donor. Galactinol consists of a galactosyl residue linked $\alpha(1 \rightarrow 1)$ to *myo*-inositol.

$$UDP\text{-}Gal + myo\text{-}inositol \rightarrow UDP + galactinol$$
$$sucrose + galactinol \rightleftharpoons raffinose + inositol$$
$$raffinose + galactinol \rightleftharpoons stachyose + inositol$$
$$stachyose + galactinol \rightleftharpoons verbascose + inositol$$

Lactose

Lactose (figure 1.11) is the main carbohydrate present in the milk of most mammals and is synthesized nearly exclusively by lactating mammary gland. It has never been found elsewhere in the animal kingdom, and occurs only very rarely in plants. In milk, it occurs in fairly high concentrations (4.5% in cows' milk, 7% in human milk), and because milk is the only food taken by newborn mammals, lactose is the main carbohydrate available to such neonates.

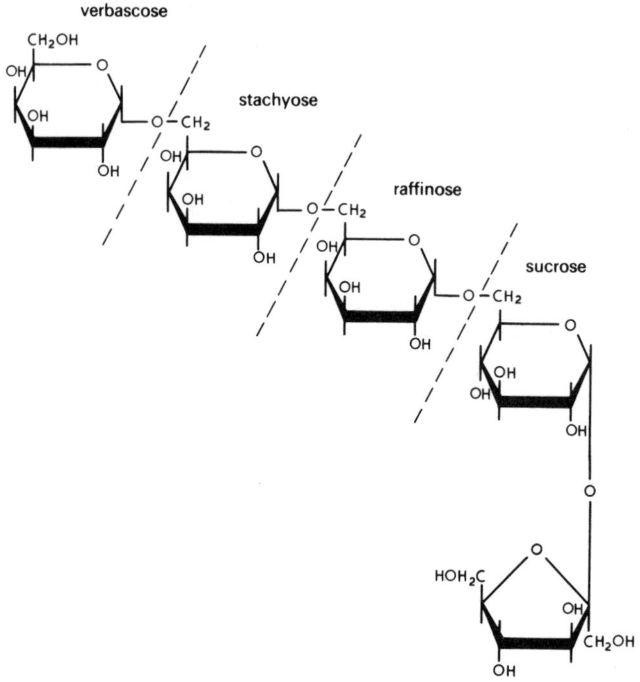

Figure 6.3   Structures of the raffinose group of oligosaccharides.

Lactose is synthesized by a galactosyltransferase present in lactating mammary gland which catalyses the transfer of galactose from UDP-galactose directly to free glucose:

$$\text{UDP-Gal} + \text{Glc} \rightarrow \text{UDP} + \text{lactose } (\text{Gal}\beta(1 \rightarrow 4)\text{Glc})$$

Unlike the synthesis of trehalose and sucrose a disaccharide-phosphate is not an intermediate.

Galactosyltransferase is a rather unusual enzyme in that its acceptor specificity depends on the presence of a protein component of milk known as α-lactalbumin. In the absence of α-lactalbumin, the K_m of the enzyme for glucose is very high (1.4 M), so that at physiological concentrations of glucose of below 1 mM the rate of lactose synthesis is insignificant. The enzyme will, however, catalyse the transfer of galactose from UDP-galactose onto terminal N-acetylglucosamine residues of glycoproteins. In the presence of α-lactalbumin, the affinity of the enzyme for glucose is considerably increased, so that the enzyme can then synthesize lactose rapidly at physiological concentrations of substrate. The enzyme is therefore a galactosyltransferase whose acceptor specificity can be varied according to the concentration of α-lactalbumin present.

This property of the enzyme seems to be important in the physiological regulation of lactose synthesis. Before birth of the young, the mammary glands of the mother contain lactose synthase in readiness for milk secretion, but little lactose is made because of a lack of α-lactalbumin. At birth, hormonal changes occur which stimulate α-lactalbumin synthesis, and therefore stimulate synthesis of lactose.

During digestion of lactose in the mammalian gut, the disaccharide is first hydrolysed to its component monosaccharides, and these are then absorbed as described on p. 89. Human infants normally have adequate levels of lactase to hydrolyse all of the lactose in their diet, but many adult non-Europeans lack the enzyme. If milk is given to such individuals, the lactose passes through the gut unabsorbed, and causes the stools to be watery due to the osmotic effect of the lactose. Lactose is also a good substrate for fermentation by intestinal microorganisms, so quantities of carbon dioxide are produced. The symptoms can be prevented by avoiding foods containing lactose.

Glycosides

Glycoside derivatives of a wide range of different compounds occur in nearly all plants and animals. The chemical properties of the aglycone component are affected by combination with carbohydrate and, in particular, the water solubility of the glycoside is usually higher than that of the aglycone. Where the aglycone has some physiological activity (e.g. hormonal or toxic activities), the glycoside derivative is generally inactive or less active than the parent compound. This provides a mechanism for regulation of the activity of the aglycone—it can be inactivated by glycosylation or, alternatively, it can be accumulated in an inactive form as the glycoside, to be released by hydrolysis in response to an appropriate stimulus.

Glycosides of plants and microorganisms

Although glycosides are of very wide occurrence in plants, their functions are still largely obscure. They are often considered to be "secondary metabolites", that is, compounds not essential to the life of the organism. Some are characteristic of only certain plant families, and have been used

by plant biologists as an aid to taxonomy. Glycosides are often responsible for the characteristic taste and smell of plants; for example, the
mustard oils (figure 6.1) are a group of thioglycosides produced by plants
of the Cruciferae family, and are responsible for the species-specific odour
of such plants.

A number of plant glycosides have profound physiological effects on
mammals, and some have been employed in this role for thousands of
years. Examples include those used for arrow poisons by native tribes of
Africa and South America, and the so-called cardiac glycosides which
have an effect on the mammalian heart. Some glycosides of the latter
group (such as those extracted from the foxglove, digitalis) are used
medically in certain types of heart disease to increase the strength of the
heart beat and slow the rate of beating. The aglycones of such glycosides
are often convulsive poisons.

Some plant glycosides are used experimentally in biochemical experi-

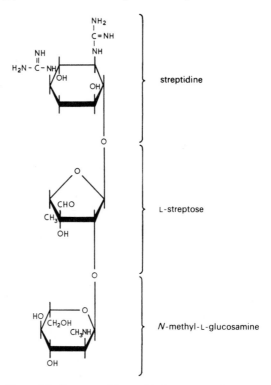

Figure 6.4   Structure of the antibiotic streptomycin.

ments as specific inhibitors. Thus phloridzin (figure 6.1) is widely used as an inhibitor of glucose transport, and ouabain (figure 6.1) as an inhibitor of the sodium/potassium ATPase of plasma membranes.

Microorganisms, in particular actinomycetes, produce a number of secondary metabolites. Some of these are glycosides and, of particular interest, some are antibiotics. Perhaps the best known of these is streptomycin (figure 6.4) in which three unusual components, N-methyl L-glucosamine, L-streptose (a branched chain sugar) and streptidine (a *scyllo*-inositol derivative containing two guanidyl groups) are linked together glycosidically. Streptomycin is an inhibitor of bacterial protein synthesis and has been the main antibiotic to be successful against tuberculosis.

Animal glycosides

Animals have the ability to inactivate and excrete compounds which have toxic or pharmacological effects. Some compounds of this type are derived directly from the food, either inadvertently or deliberately, as when drugs are administered. Others, such as steroid hormones, may be synthesized within the body to carry out some essential function, but must be rendered inactive once their job has been done. One of the most common mechanisms for modifying and inactivating such compounds is by "conjugating" them with carbohydrate. In mammals, the conjugates are glycosides of glucuronic acid, whereas insects synthesize glucosides.

In mammals, conjugation occurs primarily in the liver, but also takes place in other tissues, including the kidney and intestine. These tissues contain a glucuronyl transferase or, more probably, a mixture of glucuronyl transferases of different acceptor specificities. The glycosyl donor for these reactions is UDP-glucuronate, and acceptors include a wide range of aromatic and aliphatic compounds with one or more suitable functional groups such as $-OH$, $-NH_2$, $=NH$, $-SH$ or $-COOH$.

The effect of conjugation with glucuronic acid on the chemical properties of the aglycones is to produce a more water-soluble compound which has a negative charge due to the ionized carboxylate group. Toxic compounds are usually rendered less toxic, and are more readily excreted by virtue of the increased solubility and charged group. The route of excretion varies according to the animal species and molecular weight of the compound. In general, small-molecular-weight compounds are excreted via the kidney and urine, whereas larger compounds are excreted in the bile, and hence the faeces.

Glycosides may also be employed as chemical protective groups, to prevent a reaction occurring until the appropriate time. In this way, an inactive precursor can be accumulated in large quantities in readiness for some physiological event. An example of this is in the formation of the cockroach egg case (oötheca). The female cockroach possesses two dissimilar colleterial glands. The left gland secretes a soluble protein, a diphenoloxidase and the β-glucoside of 3,4-dihydroxybenzoate. The right gland secretes a β-glucosidase. No reaction occurs within the secretions of the left gland, because the diphenoloxidase cannot act on the 3,4-dihydroxybenzoate which is present in the protected β-glucoside form. The secretions of the two glands meet at the site of egg-case formation, and here a series of reactions is started by hydrolysis of the β-glucoside by the β-glucosidase from the right gland. The free 3,4-dihydroxybenzoate released is now a substrate for the diphenoloxidase, and is oxidized to a chemically active quinone. This in turn reacts with the protein to form cross-links with the side-chain $-NH_2$ and other groups to give an insoluble tanned protein which forms the main structural component of the finished egg case.

CHAPTER SEVEN

STORAGE POLYSACCHARIDES

When the supply of carbohydrate to an organism exceeds the rate of utilization, the surplus carbohydrates are converted into storage polysaccharides. These can be used at a later stage when the supply of carbohydrates becomes restricted. Formation of storage polysaccharides occurs typically in animals after feeding, or in green plants during photosynthesis. Microorganisms, too, can synthesize storage polysaccharides, expecially if they are grown in carbohydrate-rich media where the growth rate is restricted by limiting the concentration of an essential nutrient such as phosphate.

The advantages to the cell of storing carbohydrate as polysaccharides rather than monosaccharides lie in the physical properties of the molecules. Large quantities of free sugars would produce a high osmotic pressure within the cell and would increase the uptake of water. There is no such problem with the insoluble and osmotically-inactive polysaccharides. Most cells, in fact, maintain a rather low internal concentration of free monosaccharides by converting them to phosphates and other metabolites as soon as they enter the cell. This is important in maintaining a "downhill" concentration gradient for sugar transport into cells (see chapter 5).

One of the requirements of storage polysaccharides is that they should be capable of rapid synthesis during periods of plentiful carbohydrate supply, and that they should be capable of rapid breakdown in response to energy requirements of the organism. To permit rapid metabolism, most storage polysaccharides are deposited within the cell as roughly globular structures in which the polysaccharide chains have many loose ends available for enzyme action. In some plants this is achieved by having short simple polysaccharide chains, such as occur in inulin (p. 128).

However, in nearly all animals, and in many plants and microorganisms, this structure is achieved by having large polysaccharide molecules which are branched many times to give an open tree-like structure with many ends available to enzymes. This arrangement is characteristic of glycogen and starch, and the frequency of its occurrence in the animal and plant kingdoms suggests that it represents the optimum design for a storage polysaccharide.

The enzymes of polysaccharide synthesis and breakdown are often found loosely bound to the insoluble polysaccharides. Indeed, this association between enzyme and substrate is sometimes used as a basis for the isolation of such enzymes. It is probable that the association is of physiological importance in promoting rapid metabolism of the poly-saccharides when required.

Glycogen

Glycogen is the main storage polysaccharide of animals and of some microorganisms. In glycogen, chains of glucose residues are joined together by $\alpha(1 \rightarrow 4)$ glucosidic linkages. In addition, a smaller proportion (usually about 8–10% of the total) of $\alpha(1 \rightarrow 6)$ linkages is present, and it is these which form the branch points in the molecule. This basic structure is shown in figure 7.1.

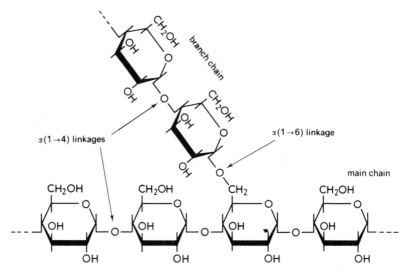

Figure 7.1 Linkage of glucose residues in glycogen.

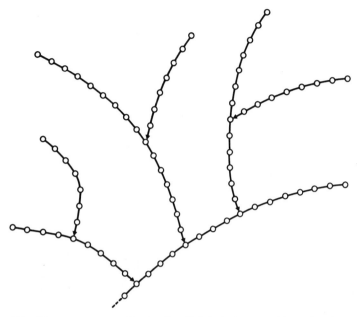

Figure 7.2 Glycogen structure. O—O α(1 → 4) linked glucose residues; O→O α(1 → 6) linked glucose residues.

The glycogen macromolecule is very large and may contain over a million glucose residues. Many α(1 → 4) linked chains are present, and multiple rebranching occurs (figure 7.2). There is one reducing end per macromolecule in which the terminal glucose unit is either unsubstituted at carbon 1 or linked to protein. All the other terminal glucose units are non-reducing with a free hydroxyl group at carbon 4 and with carbon 1 glycosidically linked to the next glucose residue. The main enzymes of glycogen synthesis and breakdown in the cell (glycogen synthase and phosphorylase) use these non-reducing chain ends as substrates.

In animal cells, glycogen is deposited in the form of particles (figure 7.3). These can be isolated from homogenates of glycogen-rich tissues such as liver, and can then be studied by electron microscopy. Such studies show the presence of large α-particles (100–150 nm in diameter) which have a rosette-like structure made up from a number of smaller β-particles approximately 25 nm in diameter. Phosphorylase and glycogen synthase are found to be associated with the glycogen particles after they have been isolated from tissues by careful procedures.

The molecular weight of glycogen molecules varies considerably, depending on the animal species, the type of tissue, and the physiological state of the animal. Even within a tissue the glycogen molecules are polydisperse, that is, they have a wide range of molecular weights. The glycogen of rat liver has molecular weights in the range 1 to 5×10^8, whereas that from rat muscle has a rather low molecular weight of about 5×10^6 and is less polydisperse.

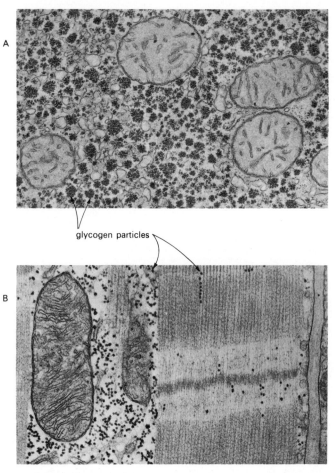

Figure 7.3 Electron micrographs of (A) liver and (B) heart muscle to show glycogen particles ($\times 33\,000$). Original micrograph by courtesy of Dr. D. W. Fawcett, Department of Anatomy, Harvard Medical School.

Glycogen biosynthesis

Two enzymes are required for glycogen synthesis. One ("glycogen syn-thase") is responsible for formation of the $\alpha(1 \to 4)$ linkages and the second ("branching enzyme") forms the $\alpha(1 \to 6)$ branch points.

Glycogen synthase (UDP-D-glucose:glycogen 4-α-D—glycosyl-trans-ferase) catalyses the transfer of glucose from UDP-glucose onto a non-reducing terminal glucose residue of a glycogen molecule:

$$\text{UDP-Glc} + [\text{glucose}]_n \to \text{UDP} + [\text{glucose}]_{n+1}$$

It is specific for the formation of the main $\alpha(1 \to 4)$ linkages of glycogen, and its action is therefore to bring about chain extension by one unit at a time (figure 7.4). Repeated transfers of glucose residues from UDP-glucose will cause elongation of the outer chains of the glycogen molecule.

The best acceptor for the glucosyl transfer reaction is the glycogen molecule itself. Smaller oligosaccharides can also act as acceptors, but give slower reaction rates than for glycogen. This requirement for a preformed polymer, or "primer" to act as an acceptor is a common feature of many enzymic reactions for synthesis of polysaccharides. There is also

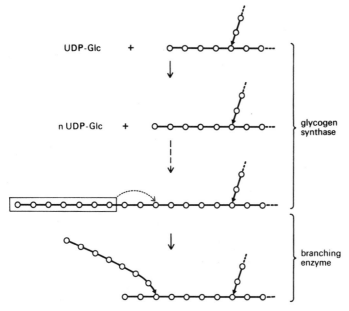

Figure 7.4 Enzymic reactions of glycogen synthesis.

evidence that protein can act as a primer for glycogen synthesis, and glycogen so formed would actually be a glycoprotein.

The second enzyme required for glycogen synthesis is "branching enzyme" ((1 → 4)-α-D-glucan:(1 → 4)-α-D-glucan 6-glucosyltransferase). This forms the α(1 → 6) linkages of the branch points by transferring part of an outer chain onto the 6 position of a glucose residue further into the molecule (figure 7.4). The acceptor glucose residue may either be in the same chain as the transferred section, or may be in an adjacent chain. The optimum chain length of the transferred section is about seven glucose residues long. In the action of branching enzyme, there is no *net* synthesis of glycosidic linkages; rather the enzyme acts by rearranging the structure of the molecule and by forming the α(1 → 6) linkages at the expense of α(1 → 4) linkages.

Glycogen breakdown

There are two general mechanisms for the breakdown of both glycogen and starch. One mechanism involves hydrolysis of the polysaccharides to give glucose as the final product. This is characteristically an extracellular process, such as occurs in the alimentary canal during digestion of food. The free glucose is transportable; it can be absorbed, transported round the body in the blood, and eventually taken up into cells. The second mechanism for glycogen breakdown involves phosphorolysis of the polysaccharide to give glucose 1-phosphate as the major product. This is characteristically an intracellular process, and the product is not transportable but is trapped within the cell. An advantage of phosphorolysis is that the glycogen is converted directly to sugar phosphate without the intervention of hexokinase and consequent use of ATP.

The intracellular process

Phosphorylase ((1 → 4)-α-D-glucan:orthophosphate glucosyltransferase) catalyses the reaction:

$$[\text{glucose}]_n + \text{Pi} \rightleftharpoons [\text{glucose}]_{n-1} + \text{Glc-1-}P$$

Glucose units linked α(1 → 4) are removed one at a time from the non-reducing ends of the glycogen molecule (figure 7.5). In this respect, the substrate specificity resembles that of glycogen synthase. Indeed, phosphorylase can be used experimentally to *extend* chains in glycogen or starch. The reaction is thermodynamically reversible, so polysaccharide synthesis occurs with high concentrations of glucose 1-phosphate and low concentrations of inorganic phosphate.

Phosphorylase removes glucose residues from the outer chains of glycogen until four glucose residues remain external to an $\alpha(1 \rightarrow 6)$ linkage. Action of phosphorylase alone on glycogen gives a "phosphorylase limit dextrin". Further breakdown requires the presence of "debranching enzyme" which has two different catalytic functions in the same protein molecule. The first is a transferase $((1 \rightarrow 4)$-α-D-glucan:$(1 \rightarrow 4)$-α-D-glucan 4-α-D-glucosyltransferase) which removes a short (optimum three residues) $\alpha(1 \rightarrow 4)$-linked chain from attachment to an $\alpha(1 \rightarrow 6)$ linked glucose and transfers it to an adjacent non-reducing

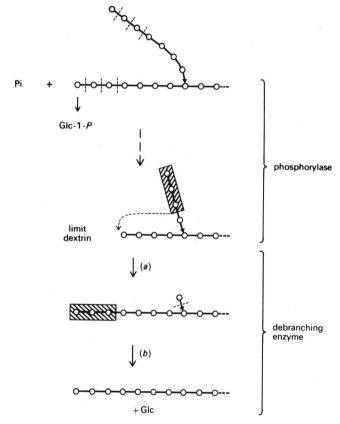

Figure 7.5 Intracellular breakdown of glycogen. The debranching enzyme has two activities: (a) transferase and (b) glucosidase.

end of the "main chain" (figure 7.5). The single $\alpha(1 \rightarrow 6)$ linked glucose residue is thus exposed by the transferase action. The second enzymic activity, amylo$(1 \rightarrow 6)$-α-D glucosidase, now hydrolyses the $\alpha(1 \rightarrow 6)$ linkage to release free glucose. The debranched chain can act as substrate for further phosphorylase action. The final products of the intracellular breakdown of glycogen are about 92% glucose 1-phosphate from phosphorolysis of the $\alpha(1 \rightarrow 4)$ linkages and about 8% glucose from hydrolysis of the $\alpha(1 \rightarrow 6)$ linkages.

The extracellular process

The extracellular digestion of glycogen and starch is a two-stage process. The first stage is hydrolysis to give maltose plus small-molecular-weight oligosaccharides. This is catalysed by α-amylase $((1 \rightarrow 4)$-α-glucan 4-glucanhydrolase), found in the saliva and pancreatic secretions of

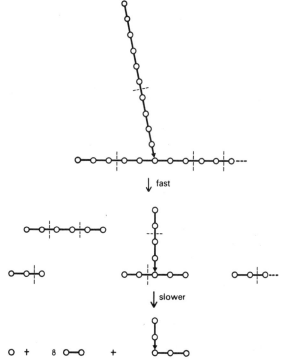

Figure 7.6   Hydrolysis of glycogen and amylopectin by α-amylase.

mammals. α-Amylase specifically hydrolyses $\alpha(1 \rightarrow 4)$ linkages, and it can attack not only the outer chains of glycogen but also the inner chains beyond the branch points. The initial action of α-amylase is to cause rapid depolymerization of glycogen to large oligosaccharides by hydrolysis of exterior and interior chains. Further hydrolysis of the large oligo-saccharides then occurs to give maltose plus small oligosaccharides containing one or more $\alpha(1 \rightarrow 6)$ linkages (figure 7.6). α-Amylase cannot hydrolyse $\alpha(1 \rightarrow 6)$ linkages of glycogen or the $\alpha(1 \rightarrow 4)$ linkages of maltose.

In the second stage of digestion, maltose and the oligosaccharides are hydrolysed to glucose by a mixture of glucosidases in the intestine. Complete hydrolysis to glucose is necessary before absorption can take place, as only monosaccharides are normally transported through animal-cell membranes. The glucosidases (maltase, isomaltase, etc.) are associated with the brush border of the mammalian intestine. This is a region of the intestinal wall which has a large surface area for absorption of products of digestion. The presence of the glycosidases in the brush border thus ensures that the final products of carbohydrate digestion are released at the site where rapid absorption can occur.

Liver and muscle glycogen

Liver and muscle contain 95% of all the glycogen in the body of mammals. The function of glycogen in these tissues is rather different. Glycogen of muscle (and many other tissues) serves as an energy reserve solely for the use of the particular cell in which it occurs. Thus the glycogen of working muscles decreases in amount when it is used to supply energy for contraction, but at the same time other non-working muscles in the body retain all of their glycogen. Liver glycogen, on the other hand, serves as a major source of blood glucose. It is of crucial importance for ensuring that glucose supply is maintained to other organs, and especially to the brain. The metabolism of liver glycogen depends very much on the nutritional state of the animal. Rapid synthesis occurs after a carbohydrate meal, and the liver glycogen is later converted back to glucose in the post-absorptive state.

In keeping with its role in supply of blood glucose, liver (and kidney) contains an enzyme, glucose 6-phosphatase, specifically responsible for converting sugar phosphates into free glucose. This enzyme is not found in muscle or in most other tissues. The overall pathways of glycogen synthesis and breakdown in liver are shown in figure 7.7.

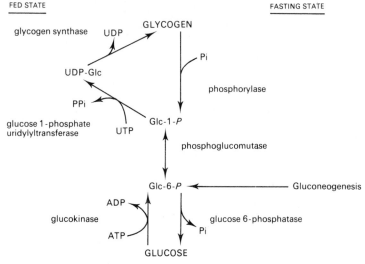

Figure 7.7   Interconversion of glucose and glycogen in liver.

Glycogen storage diseases

Our understanding of the role of different enzymes in glycogen metabolism has been helped by research into the glycogen storage diseases. These are rare diseases which arise as a result of a genetic defect in the ability of an individual to synthesize one or other of the enzymes of glycogen metabolism. For most of these diseases, the biochemical implications of the lack of an enzyme correlate well with the proposed role of the enzyme in metabolism (table 7.1). Type II disease requires further comment, however. In this disease, the glycogen which accumulates in the tissue is in two forms—one is the normal type of glycogen particle, but the other is an abnormal massive accumulation of glycogen in vesicles. It is believed that these vesicles represent lysosomes which have become gradually swollen with glycogen which they are unable to hydrolyse because of the absence of an α-glucosidase. This finding implies that in normal individuals glycogen breakdown can take place by a hydrolytic (lysosomal) mechanism, as well as by the phosphorylase pathway.

Starch

Starch is the storage polysaccharide of most plants. It consists of a mixture of two similar polysaccharides of glucose—the unbranched

Table 7.1 The glycogen storage diseases

Type	Defective enzyme	Tissue affected	Biochemical implications
I	glucose 6-phosphatase	liver	Glycogen breakdown to glucose impaired. Liver glycogen high, blood glucose low during fasting. Liver does not respond to glucagon by releasing glucose.
II	α-glucosidase of lysosomes	most tissue	Glycogen accumulates in tissues.
III	debranching enzyme	liver, sometimes muscle	Glycogen is similar to phosphorylase limit dextrin, especially after fasting. Hypoglycaemia due to impaired ability to mobilize liver glycogen.
IV	branching enzyme	liver	Glycogen has a low degree of branching.
V	phosphorylase	muscle	Impaired ability to exercise. Muscle glycogen high. No increase of lactate in blood during exercise.
VI	phosphorylase kinase	liver	Impaired ability to use liver glycogen.
VII	phosphofructokinase	muscle	Similar to Type V.

amylose and the branched-chain amylopectin. In the starch of most plants, there is about 20–25 % amylose and 75–80 % amylopectin, but this ratio is not fixed and can vary in different plant species and at different growth stages. The extremes of this variation are found in the starch from waxy varieties of maize (corn) which has virtually no amylose, and in the starch from a genetic variant of peas which has 70 % amylose.

Plants deposit starch in the form of granules, the shapes of which are characteristic of the plant species. Starch granules in "long term" storage tissues such as potato tubers are large (up to 100 μm in diameter) and may constitute a large proportion of the total tissue weight. Here the starch is laid down over a period of several months, and may then remain virtually unchanged until the following season, when it is used to provide substrates for new growth. The starch reserve of seeds is another long-term store. Seeds may remain dormant for years, but once germination starts, the starch is used within a few days.

Starch is also found in leaves, where it comprises only about 1 % of the dry weight of the tissue. Here it forms a much more temporary store of carbohydrate made by photosynthesis during daylight. At night, the starch is converted back to sugars and transported to non-photosynthetic tissues. In leaves, the granules are much smaller (about 1 μm in diameter) than in long-term storage tissues and are formed within the chloroplast where photosynthesis occurs.

When starch granules are heated in water, they swell, take up water, and gelatinize. After further heating, a colloidal solution of starch is formed. The amylose component can be separated from such solutions by addition of organic compounds such as *n*-butanol or thymol. The amylose slowly precipitates out as a complex with the organic molecule, leaving the amylopectin in solution.

Amylose

Amylose molecules consist of a thousand or more glucose residues joined through $\alpha(1 \rightarrow 4)$ linkages. Recent evidence suggests that there may also be a very small proportion of $\alpha(1 \rightarrow 6)$ linkages. The near-absence of branch points in the molecules allows them to take up a more regular conformation than is possible with the branched-chain structures of glycogen and amylopectin.

The conformation of amylose has been studied in complexes between amylose and iodine, or between amylose and organic molecules such as *n*-butanol. In such complexes, the conformation of amylose is stabilized by the presence of the complexing molecules, so that all of the molecules are in the same form and can be used to give meaningful X-ray diffraction patterns. Rundle and his colleagues were the first to carry out such studies, and were able to establish that such amylose complexes are in a helical conformation, with six glucose residues per turn of the helix. However, it is probable that in aqueous solution, amylose exists in a much looser random coil structure. The complex of amylose with iodine has an intense blue colour, and the ability to give such a colour is the basis of the iodine test for starch. The amylose-iodine complex consists of an amylose helix within which is included a linear polyiodine–iodide chain.

Amylopectin

The basic structure of amylopectin closely resembles that of glycogen. Both polymers have $\alpha(1 \rightarrow 4)$ linked glucose chains branched by $\alpha(1 \rightarrow 6)$ linkages. The most obvious difference between them is that amylopectin has a lower degree of branching than glycogen. In amylopectin, $\alpha(1 \rightarrow 6)$ linkages comprise only about 4–5 % of the total glycosidic linkages, giving an average chain length of twenty to twenty-five glucose residues, although this can vary somewhat between different plant species. There is some evidence that the branching in amylopectin is not regular, but that there may be regions of dense branching. An asymmetrical cluster structure has been suggested which could fit better than a globular structure with the physical properties of amylopectin.

The branch points of amylopectin contribute significantly to the physical properties of the macromolecule. Unlike amylose, the chains in amylopectin are interrupted by the branching, and are unable to take up helical conformations of sufficient length to associate well with organic solvents or with iodine. Thus amylose will complex approximately 20% of its own weight of iodine, whereas amylopectin complexes less than 1% iodine and gives a red-violet colour which is much less intense than that of the amylose-iodine complex.

Starch biosynthesis

Starch is synthesized by similar enzymes to those involved in glycogen synthesis in animals. The main enzyme is starch synthase (ADP-D-glucose:$(1 \rightarrow 4)$-α-D-glucan 4-α-glucosyltransferase) which catalyses the transfer of glucose from either ADP-glucose or UDP-glucose onto external chains of primer to give chain elongation through $\alpha(1 \rightarrow 4)$ linkages. Most of the synthases isolated from plants have a higher affinity for ADP-glucose as glucosyl donor than for UDP-glucose, and it is believed that it is ADP-glucose which is the normal precursor in most plants.

In non-photosynthetic tissues, the carbohydrate substrate for starch synthesis may be supplied in the form of sucrose. This can give starch by the following sequence of reactions:

$$\text{sucrose} + \text{UDP} \rightleftharpoons \text{UDP-Glc} + \text{fructose} \quad \text{(sucrose synthase)}$$

$$\text{UDP-Glc} + \text{PPi} \rightleftharpoons \text{Glc-1-}P + \text{UTP} \quad \text{(glucose-1-phosphate uridylyl transferase)}$$

$$\text{Glc-1-}P + \text{ATP} \rightleftharpoons \text{ADP-Glc} + \text{PPi} \quad \text{(glucose-1-phosphate adenylyl transferase)}$$

$$\text{ADP-Glc} + [\text{glucose}]_n \rightarrow \text{ADP} + [\text{glucose}]_{n+1} \quad \text{(starch synthase)}$$

$$\text{UTP} + \text{ADP} \rightleftharpoons \text{ATP} + \text{UDP} \quad \text{(nucleoside diphosphate kinase)}$$

Such a pathway has been found to occur in developing pea and wheat seeds. It has the advantage that there is no overall utilization of ATP because, in effect, the potential energy of hydrolysis of the glycosidic linkage in sucrose is used in the synthesis of the glycosidic linkage of starch.

Formation of the branch points during amylopectin synthesis is catalysed by the same type of transfer enzyme as for the branching enzyme of glycogen synthesis. The action of the plant enzyme (sometimes known as "Q enzyme") is such that it acts on longer chains and transfers longer sections than the corresponding enzyme from animals.

At present, it is not at all certain how the amylose and amylopectin are formed as separate populations of molecules within the same starch granule. One possibility is that separate enzyme complexes are responsible for synthesis of the two polysaccharides. According to this theory a synthase-branching enzyme complex would synthesize amylopectin, whereas amylose would be synthesized by a synthase alone. Different nucleoside diphosphate sugar precursors may be used for synthesis of the two polysaccharides and, in support of this idea, is the observation that waxy cereal grains that are virtually devoid of amylose are unable to use UDP-glucose as a precursor. The starch granule grows by addition onto the outside and, as a result, the molecules of product are probably arranged perpendicularly to the surface.

Starch breakdown

Plants are able to use both phosphorolytic and hydrolytic mechanisms for starch breakdown. Many plant tissues seem to contain both phosphorylases and amylases, and the relative physiological roles of the two processes is rather less clear-cut than for glycogen breakdown in animals; for example, plant leaves may contain sufficient activities of both types of enzyme to account for the known rates of starch breakdown. However, recent experiments by Stitt, Bulpin and ap Rees, in which homogenates of pea leaves were fractionated to isolate the chloroplasts, showed that of the starch-degrading enzymes only phosphorylase was present in the chloroplasts in sufficient amounts to account for the rate of starch breakdown. This is evidence that in chloroplasts a phosphorolytic mechanism is involved in starch breakdown.

In some germinating seeds, the hydrolytic mechanism is most important, and this may be related to the fact that in such seeds most of the starch reserves are stored outside the growing embryo (e.g. in the endosperm) and that the products of starch digestion have to be transported to the embryo. As discussed earlier (p. 112), carbohydrates are most readily transported as the neutral sugars.

The process of starch breakdown during germination has been particularly well studied in cereal seeds such as barley and rice. In barley, the starchy endosperm is surrounded by a thin layer of cells called the *aleurone layer*, and it is these cells which bring about the breakdown of the starch reserves of the endosperm. Two amylases are involved: β-amylase is already present in an inactive form before germination begins and is converted to an active form during germination, whereas α-amylase is synthesized *de novo* by the aleurone cells after germination starts and is secreted into the endosperm.

The α-amylase of plants has a similar action pattern to that of the α-amylase of animals, that is, it hydrolyses $\alpha(1 \rightarrow 4)$ linkages of both exterior and interior chains in the amylopectin to give a mixture of maltose . and small-molecular-weight oligosaccharides. β-Amylase $((1 \rightarrow 4)$-α-D-glucan maltohydrolase) is an exoenzyme which hydrolyses alternate $\alpha(1 \rightarrow 4)$ linkages to give maltose. Unlike α-amylase, it attacks the external chains of amylopectin only, and cannot by-pass the branch points to attack the interior chains. The products of exhaustive hydrolysis of amylopectin by β-amylase are maltose and a high-molecular-weight "limit dextrin" with two or three glucose residues external to the branch points. The $\alpha(1 \rightarrow 6)$ links can be hydrolysed by another enzyme (amylopectin 6-gluconohydrolase, also known as limit dextrinase or R-enzyme) specific for this type of linkage. Unlike the debranching enzyme of animals, this enzyme does not possess transferase activity. Its action is to remove short chains of two or more glucose residues from the branch points of the substrate by hydrolysing the $\alpha(1 \rightarrow 6)$ links.

Regulation of storage polysaccharide metabolism

Enzymes for both breakdown and synthesis of the storage polysaccharides are normally found present together in cells. Mechanisms are therefore required to regulate these opposing reactions to allow metabolism to respond to physiological requirements and to prevent energetically wasteful recycling of substrate between polysaccharide and monosaccharide. Extensive studies on the regulation of glycogen metabolism in mammals has revealed a particularly sophisticated series of controls working at several different levels.

Glycogen breakdown

The phosphorylases of mammalian cells exists in two interconvertible forms, *a* and *b*. Phosphorylase *b* has a low catalytic activity (unless AMP is present in high concentration) whereas phosphorylase *a* is active even in the absence of AMP. Conversion of phosphorylase *b* to *a* is effected by phosphorylase *b* kinase which catalyses an ATP-dependent phosphorylation of a specific serine residue of the phosphorylase protein. Phosphorylase *a* is therefore the phosphorylated form of the enzyme. It can be converted back to phosphorylase *b* by a protein phosphatase. The rate of glycogen breakdown in the cell can be controlled by regulating the

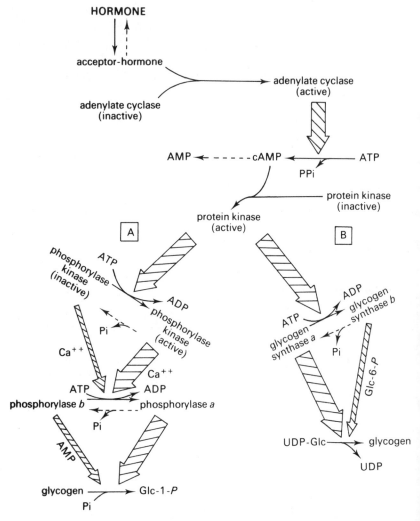

Figure 7.8 Cascade mechanisms for the hormonal regulation of glycogen metabolism. (A) Glycogen phosphorylase; (B) glycogen synthase. Hatched arrows represent the catalytic amplification stages, dotted arrows the reversal of hormone effects.

proportions of phosphorylase present in the "more active" a form and the "less active" b form. These proportions depend on the relative activities of the phosphorylase kinase and phosphatase (figure 7.8A).

It has been found that phosphorylase b kinase itself can also exist in two forms: an active phosphorylated form, and a less active dephosphorylated form. Phosphorylation is catalysed by cyclic AMP-dependent protein kinase, the activity of which requires the presence of the hormone second messenger, cyclic AMP. The concentration of cyclic AMP in the cell is, in turn, regulated by the activity of adenylate cyclase in the cell membrane. Finally, the activity of adenylate cyclase is regulated by hormones such as adrenaline or glucagon (for liver), which bind to specific receptor sites on the cell surface (see chapter 10) and activate the adenylate cyclase.

This complex series of events by which hormones can regulate glycogen breakdown is known as a "cascade" mechanism. Its complexity is dictated by a requirement to amplify the initial signal of hormone binding to receptor, and bring about the rapid breakdown of a large quantity of glycogen. (An analogy is with the multistage amplifier used to convert a weak radio wave into an electrical signal capable of operating a loudspeaker.) One molecule of hormone can activate one molecule of adenylate cyclase but, once activated, the enzyme can then catalyse the conversion of many ATP molecules to cyclic AMP. One estimate is that about 100 molecules per second of cyclic AMP are formed per active adenylate cyclase molecule. The cyclic AMP then activates an equimolar amount of protein kinase, and this in turn catalyses the phosphorylation of many molecules of phosphorylase b kinase. By the same reasoning, further amplification stages occur at the phosphorylase b to a conversion and in the final step of glycogen phosphorolysis. This gives a total of four amplification steps in the cascade, each of which may result in amplification by up to two orders of magnitude. The capacity of the system is such that one molecule of hormone could activate the breakdown of glycogen to give millions of molecules of glucose 1-phosphate. In keeping with this concept, the relative maximum activities of the enzyme are higher at the glycogen end of the cascade than at the hormone end.

It is significant that these activating reactions are all opposed by reactions which can return the system to its original state: the phosphorylated enzymes are continually being dephosphorylated; cyclic AMP can dissociate from the protein kinase and can be hydrolysed by a phosphodiesterase; hormones dissociate from their receptors and are continually being removed from the circulation. These processes allow the glycogen breakdown to return to the "resting" state once the stimulus for hormone release is removed. There is no theoretical reason why the rate of glycogen breakdown should not also be regulated through changes in these inactivating processes, and recent evidence suggests that phosphorylase phosphatase can be inhibited by a protein "Inhibitor 1" which only inhibits when phosphorylated by cyclic AMP-dependent protein kinase. This effect would reinforce the action of cyclic AMP on the cascade.

Hormonal regulation of glycogen phosphorylase occurs in liver, where glucagon regulation is of particular importance, and in muscle, where the most important hormone is probably adrenaline. Differences in response of different tissues to different hormones are partly due to the types of receptor present in the cell membranes. Thus muscle shows little or no response to glucagon, probably because there is no glucagon receptor present. However, once the adenylate cyclase has been activated, the amplification process seems to be similar in different tissues.

In muscle, there is an additional mechanism which operates independently of hormones to provide rapid activation of phosphorylase during contractions. This mechanism depends on the ability of calcium ions to activate phosphorylase kinase directly. The phosphorylase kinase then converts phosphorylase b to a, and thus promotes glycogen breakdown. This effect of calcium ions provides for rapid activation of the energy-requiring and energy-supply systems in muscle: a nerve impulse arriving at the muscle causes release of calcium ions from the sarcoplasmic reticulum, so that the concentration of calcium ions in the sarcoplasm rises from about 10^{-8} M to 10^{-6} M in a few milliseconds. The primary target of the calcium ions is the contractile system which responds by contracting, and hydrolyses ATP to provide energy for this. By activating phosphorylase b kinase, the calcium ions also trigger glycogen breakdown to provide substrate for resynthesis of the ATP by glycolysis. The efficient response of this system is shown by the fact that in resting muscle about 99% of phosphorylase is in the b form, but within one second of the onset of tetanic contractions more than 50% has been converted to the a form.

A third mechanism for the regulation of glycogenolysis in muscle is through the action of non-covalent effectors on phosphorylase, and occurs independently of protein phosphorylation. This may be the most important control under many physiological conditions. Phosphorylase b is activated by AMP and orthophosphate, and this activation is opposed by ATP and glucose 6-phosphate. Since AMP is a signal of the phosphorylation state of the adenine nucleotides in the cell (p. 40), this effect allows the phosphorylase system to respond to the requirement of the cell for ATP. A further signal may be provided by the deamination of AMP to IMP, which occurs during muscle work. Thus IMP concentrations in muscles may rise by up to 100-fold after tetanus, and IMP is an activator of phosphorylase. That such non-covalent interactions provide an effective system for control of glycogen breakdown is shown by the fact that a strain of mice which lacks phosphorylase b kinase (and therefore cannot convert phosphorylase b to a) is able to use glycogen during muscular work.

Regulation of glycogen breakdown in mammalian muscle then occurs by at least three mechanisms; one dependent on hormones, a second dependent on excitation of muscle, and a third dependent on the intracellular concentrations of nucleotides and other metabolites. Recent work from Cohen's laboratory suggests that the regulation of phosphorylase in liver may be even more complicated, and involve phosphorylation of phosphorylase b kinase at two different sites by protein kinase. The first site is phosphorylated quickly and brings about the increase in enzyme activity. The second site is phosphorylated more slowly, has no effect on enzyme activity, but promotes dephosphorylation of the first site. This allows the system to respond rapidly to hormones by an initial burst of enzyme activation in the absence of the inactivation reaction. Only later, after phosphorylation of the second site, is inactivation allowed to occur.

Glycogen synthesis

The rate of glycogen synthesis is regulated by the activity of glycogen synthase. Like phosphorylase, glycogen synthase exists in two interconvertible forms of which the a form is more active than the b form. (These are sometimes known as the "I" and "D" forms respectively). Unlike phosphorylase, however, the b form is phosphorylated and the a form is dephosphorylated, so that phosphorylation results in inactivation of glycogen synthesis (figure 7.8B). Glycogen synthase a is phosphorylated by the same cyclic AMP-dependent protein kinase which is responsible for phosphorylating phosphorylase b kinase, and is dephosphorylated by the same phosphatase which acts on phosphorylase a. There is, therefore, a reciprocal relationship whereby hormones such as adrenaline, which stimulate phosphorylase activity via the cascade mechanism, also decrease glycogen synthase activity. This prevents wasteful recycling of substrate between glycogen and glucose phosphates which could occur if both enzyme systems were to be active at the same time.

Glycogen synthesis in tissues is stimulated by insulin, so the effect of insulin on glycogen metabolism is opposite to the effect of adrenaline and glucagon. Insulin has been found to increase the proportion of glycogen synthase present in the *a* form. It is not yet known how this occurs, but cyclic AMP does not seem to be involved (p. 178).

The glycogen synthesis cascade omits one of the amplification stages of the phosphorylase system, because glycogen synthase is directly phosphorylated by protein kinase. The missing step, phosphorylase *b* kinase, is the site of calcium ion involvement in phosphorylase regulation, so calcium ions are not directly involved in regulation of glycogen synthase.

Glycogen synthase is also subject to regulation by non-covalent effectors. One of these is glucose 6-phosphate which activates glycogen synthase *b* independently of phosphorylation. This activation is antagonized by ATP and orthophosphate. Glucose 6-phosphate concentrations increase in cells when glucose supplies are plentiful, and so can stimulate glycogen synthesis independently of hormone action. The glycogen content of muscle cells can also regulate glycogen synthesis, since an inverse relationship exists between the amount of synthase in the *a* form and the concentration of glycogen. This is due to the synthase binding to glycogen, which then inhibits the action of protein phosphatase in converting glycogen synthase from the *a* to *b* form.

In liver, glucose stimulates glycogen synthesis by increasing the proportion of glycogen synthase in the active *a* form. This is of physiological importance in the conversion of excess blood glucose to glycogen after a carbohydrate meal. (The effect may be mediated by inactivation of phosphorylase *a* which is itself an inhibitor of the common protein phosphatase for both enzymes.)

Starch metabolism

The regulation of starch synthesis in plants occurs at the level of the nucleoside diphosphate sugar formation rather than at the starch synthase reaction. Thus the glucose-1-phosphate adenylyl transferase from a number of different plant tissues (especially leaves) has been shown to have regulatory properties. 3-Phosphoglycerate (an intermediate in photosynthesis, p. 74) can stimulate the activity of the enzyme from spinach leaves by some eighty times. Other intermediates found to activate plant glucose-1-phosphate adenylyl transferase include phospho-

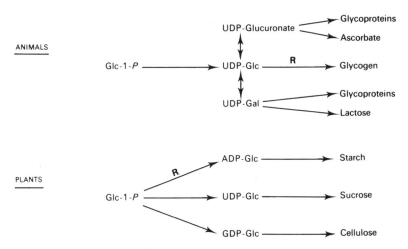

Figure 7.9 Comparative roles of nucleoside diphosphate glucose derivatives in animals and plants. R indicates the regulated step for glycogen or starch synthesis.

enolpyruvate, fructose 1,6-bisphosphate and fructose 6-phosphate, whereas inorganic orthophosphate can be a strong inhibitor.

This difference in regulatory site between the animal and plant systems may be a reflection of the rather different roles of specific nucleoside diphosphate sugars in plants (figure 7.9). In animals, UDP-glucose is involved in several different reactions, so regulation of its synthesis would affect not only glycogen synthesis but also the other reactions. Plants, however, often employ different nucleotides for different purposes, and the main fate of ADP-glucose is to provide substrate for starch synthesis. Regulation of ADP-glucose formation is then specific for the regulation of starch synthesis. The regulation of glycogen synthesis in bacteria also seems to occur at the glucose-1-phosphate adenylyl transferase reaction.

Starch breakdown in plants occurs at a slower pace than that of glycogen breakdown in animals, and the fast-acting control of enzymes by phosphorylation-dephosphorylation has not been found. Typically, regulation of starch breakdown in plants occurs by regulation of enzyme levels in the tissues. One example of this is in germinating cereal seeds where synthesis of α-amylase and activation of β-amylase is regulated by the aleurone layer in response to gibberellins (plant hormones) secreted by the embryo (p. 186). The regulation of starch breakdown in leaves may be rather faster-acting than this, so that phosphorylase activity in chloroplasts may be subject to control by as yet undiscovered factors.

Table 7.2   Examples of unusual reserve polysaccharides.

Polysaccharide	Source
Plants	
fructans (2 → 1)	Compositae (e.g. dahlia tubers)
fructans (2 → 6) and (2 → 1)	some grasses
galactomannans	Leguminosae seeds (e.g. locust bean)
galactomannans	some fungi and yeasts
xyloglucans	seeds of several families
laminarin (β(1 → 3)glucan)	some algae
Animals	
galactan	snails
mannan	locust eggs
paramylon (β(1 → 3)glucan)	some protozoa (e.g. *Euglena gracilis*)

Other storage polysaccharides

Although glycogen and starch are by far the most common storage polysaccharides, in some species other types of polysaccharide are found to have a storage function. The presence of such polysaccharides is much more common in plants than in animals (table 7.2). Only the plant fructans and galactomannans will be further dealt with here.

The fructans consist of relatively short chains of fructose residues terminating in a single glucose residue. The fructan ("inulin") of the Compositae has fructofuranose residues joined in (2 → 1) linkages. Grasses (Gramineae family) also have fructans containing (2 → 6) linkages.

Inulin can be synthesized from sucrose by transfer reactions not directly involving nucleoside diphosphate sugars. The synthesis starts by transglycosylation between two sucrose molecules catalysed by sucrose–sucrose 1-fructosyltransferase (1), then a second enzyme, fructosyltransferase (2) adds on further fructose residues one at a time from the trisaccharide Glc-Fru-Fru until a relatively small polymer of about thirty hexose residues is completed:

(1) Glc-Fru + Glc-Fru $\rightleftharpoons$ Glc-Fru-Fru + Glc

(2) Glc-Fru-Fru + Glc-Fru-Fru $\rightleftharpoons$ Glc-Fru-Fru-Fru + Glc-Fru etc.

It is not known whether alternative mechanisms exist for the synthesis of inulin via nucleoside diphosphate sugars. Although UDP-fructose has been found in dahlia and Jerusalem artichoke tubers, the presence of enzymes converting this to polysaccharides has not been established.

Galactomannans are found as storage polysaccharides in the endosperm of "albuminous" seeds from some plants of the Leguminosae family. Typically galactomannans have a main carbohydrate chain of $\beta(1 \rightarrow 4)$ linked mannose residues onto which single galactose residues are joined through $\alpha(1 \rightarrow 6)$ linkages. The frequency of substitution by galactose along the mannose chain varies according to the source of the polysaccharide.

Two functions have been suggested for the galactomannans. First, they serve as a reserve carbohydrate for growth of the new plant. Thus, during germination, hydrolytic enzymes are secreted by the aleurone layer into the endosperm, and the galactomannans are completely used within a few days. Secondly, they have the property of being able to retain water, and their presence may prevent complete desiccation of seeds exposed to high temperatures.

CHAPTER EIGHT

STRUCTURAL POLYSACCHARIDES

Most living cells are surrounded by extracellular structures which serve to protect and support them; for example, unicellular organisms such as bacteria have cell walls which may make up 20 to 30% of the dry weight of the organisms. Higher plants also have cell walls; these have the functions of protecting the individual cells, and also help to support the whole plant. Animal cells do not have walls as such, but are supported and protected by skeletons, skins and connective tissues.

Nearly all of these extracellular structures are chemically complex, and are mixtures of several different materials, each of which has a rather different function. In most structures, both proteins and carbohydrates occur, and there may be specific interactions between the two. In addition, other components are often present, for example, calcium salts occur in bones, teeth, and in crustacean exoskeletons. The detailed organization of the materials differs in individual cases, but a common arrangement is one in which strong fibres of one material are supported in a matrix of a softer material, rather as iron rods are embedded in cement to make reinforced concrete. Such an arrangement is found in plant cell walls, where the fibres are of the polysaccharide cellulose; in insect exoskeleton, where they are of another polysaccharide, chitin; and in animal connective tissues, in which the fibres are of the protein collagen.

All of these structural materials are synthesized by the cells they protect and support. Because the materials are insoluble and usually macromolecular, they pose special problems in synthesis and export from the cells, and this topic has been the subject of considerable research effort over recent years.

Although a great number of different structural materials are found in different organisms, it is proposed to focus here on just a small number of them which have been chosen because most is known of their structure, function and synthesis.

Bacterial cell walls

The interior of bacterial cells contains considerable quantities of dissolved substances (ions, metabolic intermediates, etc.) which together exert a high osmotic pressure of up to 20 atmospheres. These cell contents are separated from the external medium by the plasma membrane and, since the medium is usually hypotonic relative to the cell interior, there is a strong tendency for the cell to take up water osmotically. Without any restriction on this process, the cell would swell and burst. To prevent this, bacteria have a cell wall external to the plasma membrane which is capable of withstanding these osmotic forces.

The cell walls of bacteria are of particular interest for a number of reasons:

(1) They bear the antigenic determinants by which mammalian systems recognize them as "foreign" and are able to develop specific antibodies to counteract them.
(2) The synthesis of the cell wall is the target for the action of a number of antibiotics, in particular the penicillins.
(3) The mechanism of synthesis of the walls is an interesting biochemical system which has provided useful clues for the study of the synthesis of animal and plant extracellular structures.

Structure

Bacteria can be divided into two main groups: Gram-positive and Gram-negative, according to their ability to take up stain in the Gram reaction. Although this property appears to be rather arbitrary, it turns out that this classification divides bacteria into two groups which have a number of physiological and chemical differences. In particular, the cell wall structures of the two types are rather different.

Both groups have in common the presence of a material known as peptidoglycan, which is the main structural component of all bacterial cell walls. However, the walls contain a number of additional components, and these differ between the Gram-positive and Gram-negative bacteria. The Gram-negative bacteria are characterized by the presence of lipopolysaccharide which forms an outer membrane system external to the plasma membrane and the peptidoglycan. It is this which is presumed to prevent uptake of Gram stain. Gram-positive bacteria lack such a second membrane, but usually possess a teichoic acid or teichuronic acid component. In general, it is the additional components to the peptidoglycan which are on the outermost surface of the bacterium and which carry the antigenic determinants.

The general structure of peptidoglycan is the same for all bacteria (figures 8.1 and 8.2), although there are detailed species-specific differences in the identity of some of the amino-acid components and in the type of peptide cross-linking that occurs. The structure is built up as a network with carbohydrate chains running in one direction and peptide side-chains running in the other direction. Some, but not all, of the peptide chains are cross-linked to the peptide chains of adjacent molecules, so that the two-dimensional network is formed. In Gram-positive bacteria, there

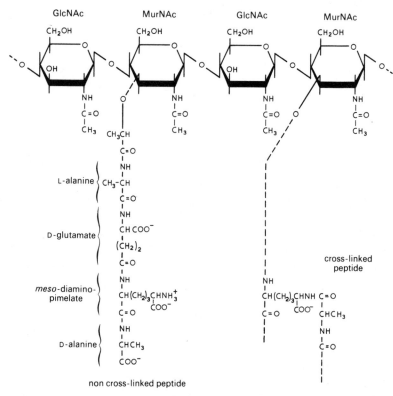

Figure 8.1 Structure of peptidoglycan. Some variation occurs in the structure of peptidoglycan in different bacterial species. In particular, in Gram-positive organisms the identity of the third amino acid (diaminopimelate above) varies with the species.

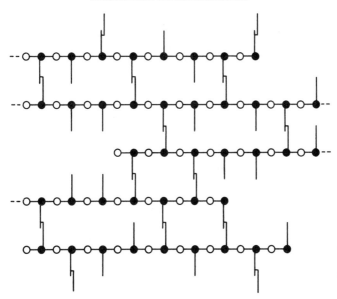

Figure 8.2 Two-dimensional structure of peptidoglycan. ● = *N*-acetylmuramate: ○ = *N*-acetylglucosamine.

are several layers of peptidoglycan with cross-linking between layers, but in most Gram-negative walls there is only one layer. The peptidoglycan completely surrounds the bacterial cell as a covalently-bound network or "bag-shaped macromolecule" which has considerable resistance to outward pressure and thus protects the cell from osmotic lysis. If the peptidoglycan is dissolved or weakened by treatment with hydrolytic enzymes such as lysozyme, the cells swell and are killed in hypotonic environments.

The carbohydrate chains of peptidoglycan consist of alternating residues of *N*-acetylglucosamine and an unusual sugar, *N*-acetylmuramate, which is only found in bacteria. These are joined by $\beta(1 \rightarrow 4)$ linkages. The peptide side-chains normally consist of four amino acids, and these alternate between residues in the L-configuration and those in the less common D-configuration. Because most peptidases specifically hydrolyse peptides containing only L-amino acids, the peptidoglycan is resistant to attack from such enzymes.

The teichoic acids of Gram-positive bacteria are built up of chains of either ribitol phosphate or glycerol phosphate. They usually carry additional species-specific components such as sugars or amino acids (figure

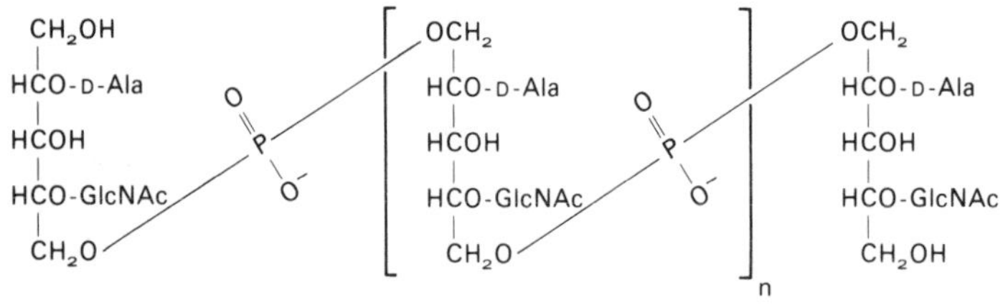

Figure 8.3 Structure of ribitol teichoic acid from cell walls of *Staphylococcus aureus*. n = 6 to 10.

8.3). An important function of teichoic acids seems to be to concentrate cations, particularly magnesium ions, in the region immediately outside the plasma membrane. At neutral pH, the phosphate groups of the teichoic acids carry negative charges which attract cations and act as ion-exchangers on the cell surface. The importance of this acidic material is seen in bacteria grown on media containing small (limiting) amounts of phosphate. Such organisms use the available phosphate for essential purposes, such as nucleic-acid synthesis, but stop making teichoic acids. Instead, they make a new component called teichuronic acid, which is a polymer containing uronic-acid residues but no phosphate. The carboxylate groups of the uronic-acid residues gives teichuronic acid the necessary negative charge so that it can functionally replace the teichoic acid.

The plasma membranes of Gram-positive bacteria also contain teichoic acids and these are always of the glycerol phosphate type. They are anchored in the membrane by a lipid-linked tail, and are sometimes known as lipoteichoic acids. It has been proposed that the membrane lipoteichoic acids function to transport Mg^{++} into the cell from the pool of ions bound to the wall teichoic acid. Lipoteichoic acids are not replaceable by teichuronic acids under conditions of phosphate limitation.

Complex polysaccharides are major components of walls of Gram-negative bacteria, and some of these are linked to lipids as lipopolysaccharides. The lipopolysaccharides of the Enterobacteriaceae have been studied in considerable detail, and the relationship between the carbohydrate structure and the antigenic behaviour of such molecules has been established. These polysaccharides are characterized by the presence of two unusual sugars in the molecule: 2-keto-3-deoxyoctonate and L-glycero-D-mannoheptose.

Some bacteria have further components external to the cell wall which take the form of capsules or of slime layers. These do not appear to be essential to the life of the organisms, since mutants lacking these components are able to grow successfully. They may function to prevent desiccation, to act as a barrier to phage attack, and to provide a charged surface. *Streptococcus mutans*, which is partly responsible for plaque formation and dental decay, produces an extracellular 1,3-glucan which enables the bacteria to stick to teeth.

Synthesis of cell walls

Synthesis of the peptidoglycan component of the cell wall takes place in three stages:

(1) Assembly of a carbohydrate-peptide unit as a uridine diphosphate derivative inside the cell.
(2) Transfer of this unit to a lipid carrier in the plasma membrane and transport through the membrane.
(3) Polymerization outside the membrane by formation of glycosidic linkages to carbo-hydrate chains and peptide bonds to cross-link the side-chains.

The first intracellular step is the synthesis of UDP-N-acetylmuramate from UDP-N-acetylglucosamine and phosphoenolpyruvate (figure 8.4). An important function of the N-acetylmuramate is to act as a link between the carbohydrate chain and the peptide, and this link is achieved in the next step by formation of an amide bond from the carboxylate group of the sugar to the amino group of L-alanine. The next series of reactions results in addition of amino acids to complete a pentapeptide side-chain. The enzymes catalysing these reactions are all specific for their particular acceptor group, as well as for the amino acid to be added, and all the reactions use ATP for synthesis of the peptide bonds. The first three amino acids are added one at a time, but the final D-alanine-D-alanine is added as a dipeptide.

The next step of the process involves transfer of the carbohydrate-pentapeptide from UDP to a lipid carrier in the plasma membrane (reaction 1, figure 8.5). The carrier is a C-55 polyisoprenol phosphate:

$$CH_3C{=}CHCH_2\left[CH_2\overset{\overset{\displaystyle CH_3}{|}}{C}{=}CHCH_2\right]_9CH_2\overset{\overset{\displaystyle CH_3}{|}}{C}{=}CHCH_2OPO_3^{-}$$

N-Acetylglucosamine is then transferred from UDP-N-acetylglucosamine to form a $\beta(1 \rightarrow 4)$ linkage with the N-acetylmuramate residue (2). The whole precursor unit is transported on the lipid carrier to the outer side of the plasma membrane (3) and polymerization can take place: a trans-glycosylase catalyses the transfer of the precursor from the lipid carrier onto a section of growing peptidoglycan in the cell wall to extend the carbohydrate chains (4). Cross-linking of the peptide chains takes place by a transpeptidation reaction in which a new peptide bond is formed between the carboxylate group of the penultimate D-alanine residue of one chain and the amino group of the third amino acid (diaminopimelate in the example of figure 8.1) in an adjacent chain (figure 8.6). This transpeptidation reaction takes place at the expense of the terminal D-alanine-

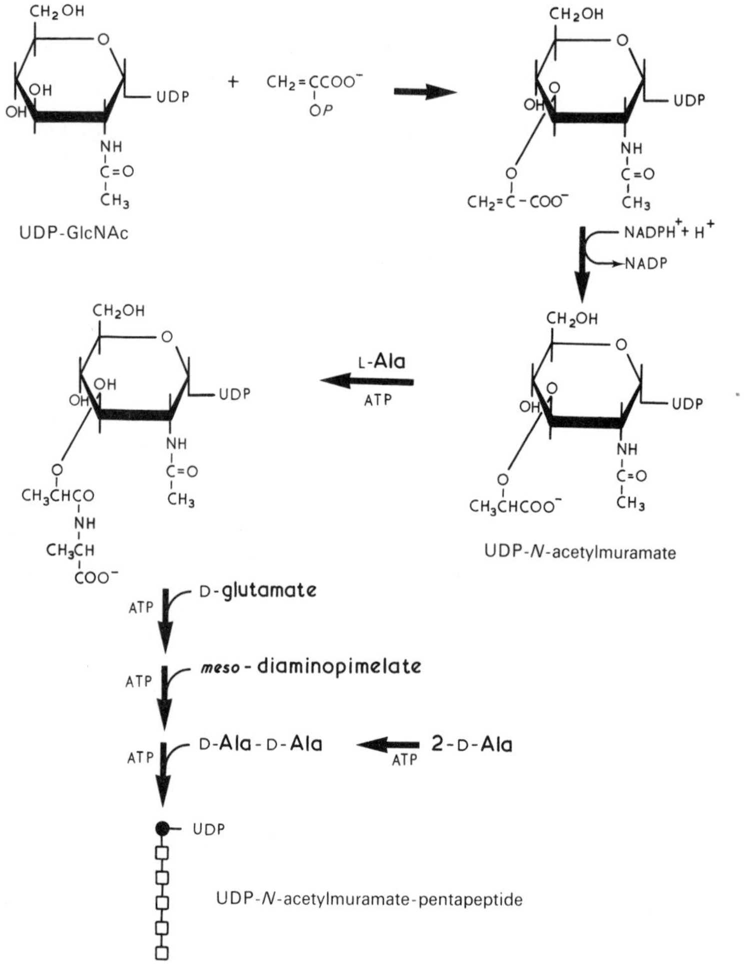

Figure 8.4 Synthesis of peptidoglycan precursor. ● = N-acetylmuramate; □ = amino acids.

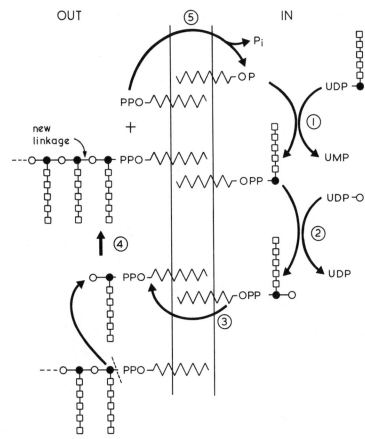

Figure 8.5 Transfer of precursor to lipid carrier, transport across the membranes and formation of glycosidic linkage. $\wedge\!\wedge\!\wedge\!\wedge\bigcirc$ = undecaprenol carrier.

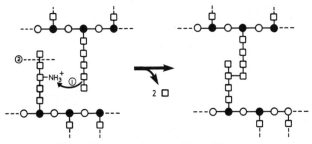

Figure 8.6 Transpeptidase (1) and carboxypeptidase (2) reactions in peptidoglycan synthesis.

D-alanine peptide bond, and can be seen as a mechanism for peptide bond synthesis in the absence of ATP. This is very necessary in the environment outside the plasma membrane where there is otherwise no energy supply for the endergonic reaction of peptide bond synthesis. In addition to the transpeptidation reaction, some of the terminal D-alanine is removed by a specific carboxypeptidase, so that in the cell wall the peptide chains contain four amino acids each, in contrast to the five of the precursors.

Growth of the bacterium has to take place within a structurally sound cell wall. To insert new material into the wall, acceptor sites are created by glycosaminidases and peptidases secreted into the wall. This must be a carefully controlled process, as too much hydrolysis could result in weakening of the peptidoglycan network. However, it is not yet known how the degradative and synthetic processes are balanced to give controlled growth in the appropriate morphological configuration for the bacterium.

Synthesis of the other cell-wall components takes place according to the same general principles outlined for peptidoglycan: assembly of precursor inside the cell, transport through the membrane on a lipid carrier, and polymerization outside the membrane. Mechanisms of this type have been shown for synthesis of cell-wall teichoic acids of Gram-positive bacteria and for the O-antigen polysaccharides of the Gram-negative Enterobacteriaceae.

Antibiotics which interfere with cell-wall synthesis

To be of medical use, antibiotics not only have to interfere with some function essential to the life of bacteria, but must do this without affecting essential functions in the host. The best targets for antibiotics are therefore those in which the affected process in the bacterium differs markedly from that in mammals. Synthesis of cell-wall peptidoglycan is one such process: it occurs by a unique reaction sequence; it involves components (N-acetylmuramate, D-amino acids) not normally found in other organisms; and it is essential to the life of the bacterium.

Table 8.1 lists some of the antibiotics known to interfere with peptidoglycan synthesis. In general, such antibiotics are only effective on growing cells (i.e. cells actively synthesizing cell wall), and kill the cells by osmotic lysis as a result of production of a weakened cell wall. Thus bacteria grown in isotonic media with penicillin are able to survive as "spheroplasts" with an incomplete cell wall because they are protected against osmotic stress by the medium.

Table 8.1   Antibiotics acting on peptidoglycan synthesis.

Antibiotic	Analogue of	Site of action
phosphonomycin	phosphoenolpyruvate	synthesis of UDP-N-acetylmuramate
D-cycloserine	D-alanine	synthesis of D-Ala and D-Ala-D-Ala
penicillins and		
cephalosporins	D-Ala-D-Ala	transpeptidase and carboxypeptidase
bacitracin	—	dephosphorylation of undecaprenol pyrophosphate
vancomycin	—	incorporation of lipid bound precursor into cell wall
tunicamycin	N-acetyl glucosamine	transfer of N-acetylglucosamine onto precursor

Two of these antibiotics are very simple molecules. D-Cycloserine is a structural analogue of D-alanine and interferes with peptidoglycan synthesis by acting as a competitive inhibitor of two enzymes—the alanine racemase which synthesizes D-alanine from its L-isomer, and D-alanine-D-alanine synthase. Phosphonomycin is also a simple molecule and is a structural analogue of phosphoenolpyruvate. It acts as an inhibitor of UDP-N-acetylmuramate synthesis by binding irreversibly to the enzyme in place of the substrate.

The penicillins and cephalosporins are a group of chemically-similar antibiotics derived from amino acids. They bind to a number of different proteins in bacterial cells, but their most important effect seems to be inhibition of the transpeptidation reaction of cell-wall cross-linking. Strominger has suggested that the penicillins are analogues of the D-alanine-D-alanine terminal peptide of the precursor, and bind to the transpeptidase in place of substrate. Penicillins also inhibit the carboxypeptidase which hydrolyses terminal D-alanine residues from non-cross-linked side-chains. When some species of bacteria are treated with penicillin, a soluble peptidoglycan-like product is formed which is defective in cross-links and has pentapeptide side-chains in place of the tetrapeptides of the normal product.

Plant cell walls

Most plant cell walls contain cellulose fibres embedded in a matrix of other materials. The matrix has a rather variable composition, but the most common components are polysaccharides, water, glycoprotein and sometimes lignin. The proportions of these vary according to the species of plant and the stage of growth.

During development, two different phases of cell-wall growth can be recognized:

(1) Primary cell-wall formation occurs during the main growth phase of the cell. The primary cell walls of different types of plant cell are all rather similar in structure and are relatively thin. They consist of cellulose fibres in a relatively soft matrix with a higher water content. This wall is sufficiently plastic to allow some flow of components during wall expansion.
(2) The secondary cell walls are formed after growth has ceased and while differentiation of the cell occurs. During this phase, considerable thickening of the walls with cellulose occurs, and lignin may also be incorporated. The wall formed at this stage is more specialized and is specific to the type of differentiated cell being formed.

Cellulose

Cellulose contains D-glucopyranose residues joined through $\beta(1 \rightarrow 4)$ linkages in unbranched chains containing 2500 to 14000 residues. The glucose residues in the chain tend to take up a preferred conformation in which the ring oxygen of one residue is hydrogen-bonded to the hydroxyl at position 3 of the next residue (figure 8.7). In the plant, cellulose molecules are assembled together in "microfibrils" which consist of bundles of 40 or more cellulose molecules arranged together in a regular pattern along the main axis of the complex. Adjacent chains are held together by hydrogen bonds between them. It is the ability of cellulose molecules to give compact and tightly packed aggregates which gives the microfibrils their high strength, insolubility and chemical inertness. The regular arrangement of cellulose molecules gives the microfibrils some crystalline regions which can be studied by X-ray diffraction. Other

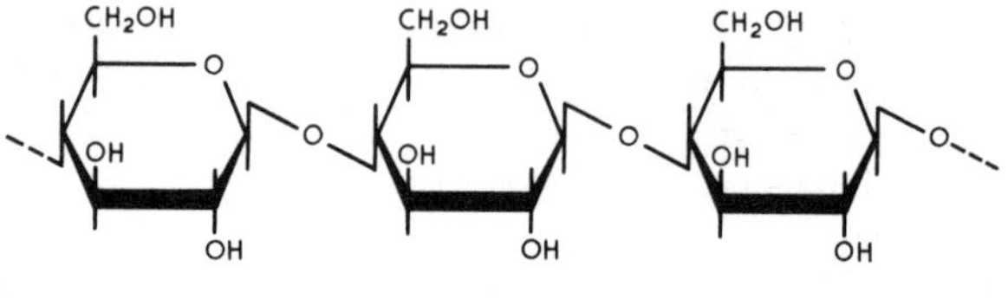

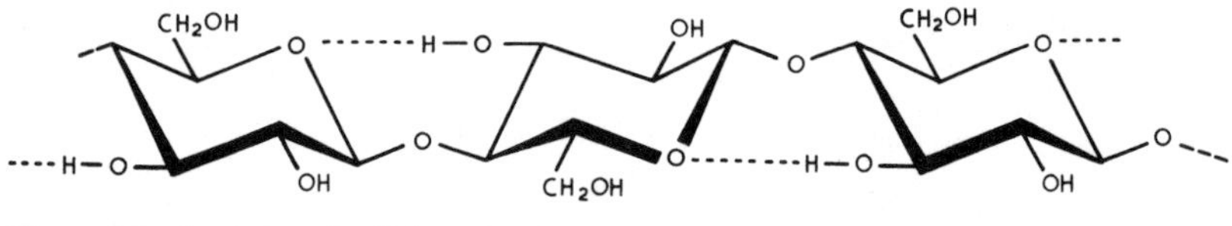

Figure 8.7 Structure of cellulose. (A) Haworth formula. (B) Conformational formula to show hydrogen bonding between the C-3 hydroxyl and the O of the ring.

Table 8.2   Matrix polysaccharides of plant cell walls.

Polysaccharide	Main chain sugars	Additional sugars
Hemicelluloses		
xyloglucan	glucose	xylose (galactose, fucose, arabinose)
arabinoxylan	xylose	arabinose
glucans	glucose	
xylans	xylose	arabinose, glucuronate
mannans	mannose	glucose, galactose
galactans	galactose	galactose, arabinose
Pectic substances		
galacturonan	galacturonate	rhamnose
arabinan	arabinose	arabinose
galactan	galactose	

regions of the microfibrils are less ordered, and there is evidence that in many species of plant a significant proportion (10% or more) of the monosaccharide residues are not glucose. It is likely that the crystalline regions of the microfibrils contain chains of the $\beta(1 \to 4)$ linked glucan, and the amorphous regions contain covalently linked sections of a different composition.

In many fungal cell walls, chitin is the main structural polysaccharide instead of cellulose. This is a polymer of N-acetylglucosamine and is also found in the arthropod exoskeleton (p. 143). Some groups of marine algae also lack cellulose, and here its structural role is taken over by a $\beta(1 \to 3)$ xylan in some species, or by a linear $\beta(1 \to 4)$ mannan in other species.

Matrix polysaccharides

Higher plants contain a number of different matrix polysaccharides. These are sometimes classified into two main groups, the hemicelluloses and the pectic substances, distinguished mainly by their differing solubilities in various reagents. The hemicelluloses can be extracted from cell walls by alkaline solutions, and pectic substances are extracted by solutions of chelating agents or by acidic solutions. Most hemicelluloses contain predominantly neutral sugars such as xylose, glucose, mannose, arabinose and galactose (table 8.2). Pectic substances are often uronic acid-containing polysaccharides, of which the most common type is a $\beta(1 \to 4)$ linked D-galacturonan. The carboxylate groups of the uronic acids are esterified to a greater or lesser extent with methyl groups. Any nonesterified carboxylate groups are negatively charged, and bind calcium or magnesium ions in the cell wall. Pectic substances may contain additional species-specific sugars glycosidically linked to some of the uronic-acid residues.

The pectic substances can form viscous sticky solutions, and play an important role in the middle lamellae between cells where they act as a cement to hold the cells together. It is these substances, too, which are solubilized from fruits during jam-making and give the final product its characteristic gel texture.

Another component of plant cell walls is a glycoprotein sometimes referred to as *extensin*. It contains peptide chains with a high proportion of the amino acid hydroxyproline. In extensin, arabinose-containing oligosaccharides are glycosidically linked to the hydroxyproline residues and, in addition, some galactose may be linked to serine residues in the protein. It is not certain what function this glycoprotein plays in the wall. One suggestion is that it has a structural function along with the matrix polysaccharides, and another suggestion is that it is involved in the synthesis of the cell wall.

Synthesis of the plant cell wall

The general process for synthesis of plant cell walls resembles in some respects the synthesis of bacterial walls: synthesis of nucleoside diphosphate sugar precursors within the cell, transport across a membrane, and polymerization outside the membrane. Additional complications exist in plant cells because the eukaryotic cell has a multiple membrane system (including plasma membrane, endoplasmic reticulum, and Golgi apparatus), and because the cellulose is assembled into microfibrils.

Synthesis of the matrix polysaccharides is believed to occur in the internal membrane system of the cell, particularly in the Golgi apparatus. This type of process is described in more detail in connection with the synthesis of extracellular polysaccharides in animals (p. 148).

The synthesis of cellulose appears to be rather different from that of the matrix polysaccharides, and probably takes place at the plasma membrane. The individual cellulose molecules have to be organized into microfibrils, and the most likely process to achieve this is one in which all of the molecules making up a microfibril are synthesized synchronously at a growing microfibril end. There is some uncertainty as to the nucleoside diphosphate glucose precursor of cellulose. There is evidence that in some plants it is GDP-glucose, but for others it could be UDP-glucose. This discrepancy may be resolved if recent work on algae by Hopp *et al.* is more generally applicable: it was shown that UDP-glucose is a precursor for synthesis of a polyisoprenol pyrophosphate glucan which could give a protein-glucan complex. The protein-glucan could then act as a primer and undergo chain extension with GDP-glucose as precursor to give a cellulose-like polymer.

A further problem in synthesis of plant cell walls is a morphological one. Plant cells usually grow in one direction (lengthways) and new wall material is added to the whole surface of the cell from the inside. Initially the cellulose microfibrils are arranged transversely, i.e. at right angles to the long axis of the cell. As the cell grows, the microfibrils are pulled round to become reoriented in the direction of growth. This is a gradual process, and the orientation will depend on the extent that growth has taken place since the microfibrils were originally laid down. Thus the outer (oldest) layers of the cell wall have microfibrils lying longitudinally, the inner layers have transverse microfibrils, and the intermediate layers have partly reoriented microfibrils. This arrangement of layers with cellulose microfibrils running in different directions gives the wall strength to resist tension in all directions.

The arthropod exoskeleton

Many invertebrates have an exoskeleton which serves for protection as a skin and also acts as a frame to maintain the shape of the animal and to provide a firm base for muscle attachment. The best-studied exoskeletons are those of the arthropods, where different examples vary from the thin cuticles of small flying insects to the thick heavily mineralized skeletons of some crustaceans.

The insect exoskeleton consists of several different layers. The outermost layer of epicuticle contains waxes which make the animal impervious to water, and thus prevents desiccation. The main bulk of the cuticle is the exo- and endocuticle which are made up largely of a mixture of roughly equal amounts of chitin and proteins. The outer layers of exocuticle are cross-linked by sclerotization. The most important structural element in the cuticle is chitin which resembles cellulose in being an unbranched polymer of $\beta(1 \rightarrow 4)$ linked sugars (figure 8.8). It differs from cellulose only in the presence of an N-acetylamido group in place of the hydroxyl group at C-2 of the sugar residues. Like cellulose, chitin molecules occur organized together in microfibrils consisting of regular arrays of molecules held together by hydrogen bonding, and this arrange-

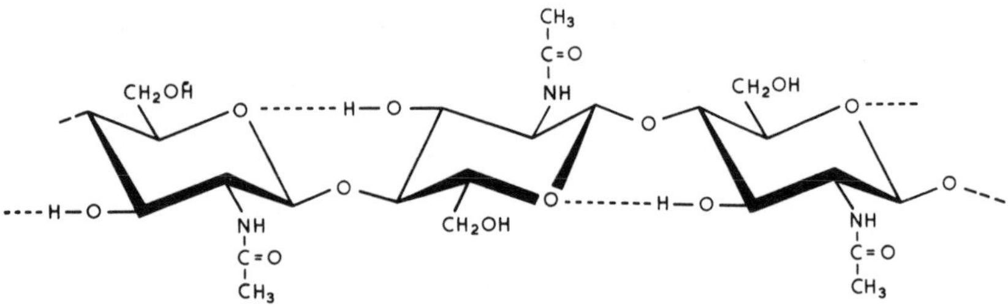

Figure 8.8   Structure of chitin.

ment gives the polymer its structural strength and resistance to chemical attack.

The epidermal cells of insects secrete chitin in daily growth layers to give lamellae of chitin sandwiched between layers of protein matrix. The direction in which the microfibrils are aligned is changed from one day to the next, to give the cuticle a plywood-like structure with strength in all directions.

The precursor for chitin synthesis in the epidermis is UDP-*N*-acetyl-glucosamine, but it is not yet known how the polymerization reaction takes place at the surface of the cells to give chitin microfibrils oriented in a given direction. The process of chitin synthesis is a target for the action of a new group of insecticides which are urea derivatives containing aromatic rings and halogens. As for antibiotics acting on bacterial cell walls, the target is a suitable one because the inhibited process does not occur in mammals, yet it is essential to the life of the attacked organism. Only immature insects are killed by these insecticides; fully grown adults with completed exoskeletons are not affected.

Mammalian connective tissues

The bony skeleton of mammals provides a framework for supporting the tissues and organs of the body. Within this framework, the connective tissues carry out other structural roles in providing an external skin for the animal, in holding the organs in their correct position, and for other more specialized functions. Connective tissues are softer than bone and provide a greater degree of flexibility. Most contain the protein collagen as a fibrous element embedded in a matrix of polysaccharides known as the acidic glycosaminoglycans. Table 8.3 gives a summary of some of these connective tissues.

Table 8.3 Glycosaminoglycans of connective tissues

Tissue	Glycosaminoglycans
cartilage	chondroitin sulphate, keratan sulphate, hyaluronate
skin	dermatan sulphate, chondroitin sulphate
synovial fluid	hyaluronate
vitreous humor (eye)	hyaluronate
cornea (eye)	keratan sulphate, chondroitin sulphate
blood vessel walls	chondroitin sulphate, heparan sulphate
lung	heparin, heparan sulphate

Table 8.4 Compositions of some acidic glycosaminoglycans

Glycosaminoglycan	Amino sugar	Uronic acid	Sulphate
hyaluronate	glucosamine	D-glucuronate	none
chondroitin sulphate	galactosamine	D-glucuronate	4-O-sulphate and/or 6-O-sulphate on galactosamine
dermatan sulphate	galactosamine	L-iduronate (D-glucuronate)	4-O-sulphate on galactosamine
heparan sulphate	glucosamine	L-iduronate (D-glucuronate)	6-O-sulphate on glucosamine some N-sulphate
heparin	glucosamine	L-iduronate (D-glucuronate)	3/6-O-sulphate on glucosamine 2-O-sulphate on iduronate N-sulphate on glucosamine
keratan sulphate	glucosamine	(galactose)	6-O-sulphate on glucosamine

Structure of glycosaminoglycans

Most of the acidic glycosaminoglycans have a repeating disaccharide unit consisting of an amino sugar and uronic-acid residue (table 8.4 and figure 8.9). The exception to this is in keratan sulphate where the uronic acid is replaced by a galactose residue. In most glycosaminoglycans, the amino sugars are present as N-acetyl derivatives, although heparin contains N-sulphate groups in place of N-acetyl groups. In all the glycosaminoglycans except hyaluronate, some of the hydroxyl groups of the amino sugars are esterified with sulphate.

Most glycosaminoglycans occur in covalent linkage with protein as "proteoglycans". This may involve a special linkage region which for chondroitin sulphate consists of a trisaccharide of neutral sugars, Gal-Gal-Xyl, glycosidically linked to a serine residue of the protein (p. 150). Often several separate glycosaminoglycan chains are found linked to the same protein chain, as in the proteoglycan component of cartilage. For hyaluronate, the evidence is that most, if not all, of the molecules are not joined to protein by covalent linkages.

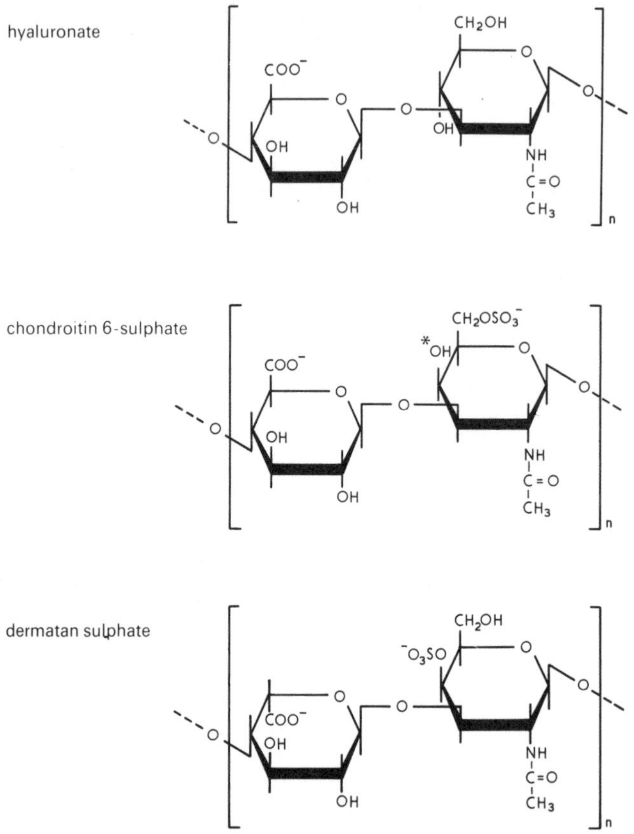

Figure 8.9 Repeating structures of some acidic glycosaminoglycans. In chondroitin 4-sulphate, the sulphate group is esterified at the position marked with an asterisk.

The presence of carboxylate and sulphate groups gives the glycosaminoglycans a high negative charge density which has a marked influence on the physicochemical properties of the molecules. Glycosaminoglycan molecules tend to take up a fairly random conformation in solution and occupy as much solvent space as is available. Because they are long polymeric molecules and are usually bound together as proteoglycans, they are liable to become partly entangled together in solution. These factors contribute to the high viscosity of solutions of glycosaminoglycans. The presence of charged anionic groups fixed to the matrix in connective tissues requires the additional presence of cations to maintain electrical neutrality. This elevates the osmotic pressure within the matrix and creates a turgor in the tissue.

The other main component of connective tissues is the structural protein collagen, which is present as fibres consisting of three collagen molecules twisted together like a rope. It is characterized by the presence of some hydroxylysine residues in the peptide chain, to which glucose and galactose are linked as disaccharide side-chains. Some connective tissues also contain another fibrous protein called *elastin*.

The physical properties of connective tissues depend both on the collagen fibres which resist stretching, and on the hydrated network of glycosaminoglycans which resist compression. The composition of different tissues varies according to their function. Such factors as the ratio of collagen to glycosaminoglycan and the type (and therefore charge density) of the glycosaminoglycan, affect the physical properties of the tissue.

One example is the vitreous humour of the eye, which is a jelly-like solution of hyaluronate. It contains no fibrous material as it must remain transparent to light. At the other extreme, tendons have a very high collagen content, and the fibres are aligned along the long axis to give flexible strength in the direction of muscle pull.

The synovial fluid acts as a lubricant at joints between bones, and this fluid contains hyaluronate as the main polysaccharide component. It is the ability of the hyaluronate to form viscous solutions which gives the synovial fluid some of its lubricating properties. In addition, the hyaluronate solutions have an elastic property which gives the tissue an ability to absorb sudden physical shocks to which joints may be subjected. In some forms of arthritis, the lubrication of the joint is impaired by a defect in the synovial fluid: if either the concentration of hyaluronate is too low, or if it is present in a partly depolymerized form, a fluid with low viscosity and poor lubricating properties results.

The organization of the macromolecular components of cartilage is known in some detail: an important unit is the proteoglycan molecule which consists of a central protein core to which chondroitin sulphate and keratan sulphate are covalently attached (figure 8.10). The molecular weight of the proteoglycan components is about 200 000, but a much larger assembly (molecular weight up to 50×10^6) is produced when several proteoglycan molecules form a complex with a long hyaluronate chain. Specific link proteins are required to join the proteoglycans to hyaluronate. The collagen fibres are embedded in this matrix and are held in place partly by non-specific electrostatic interactions between the acidic polysaccharides and basic residues on the protein, and partly by more

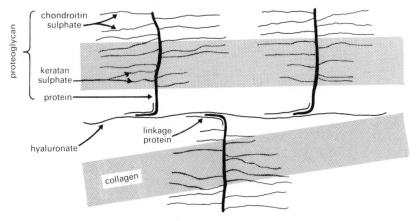

Figure 8.10   Possible arrangement of components in cartilage. Proteoglycan complexes are arranged along a hyaluronate chain to form a large aggregate, and the collagen fibres are bound ionically to the proteoglycan.

specific interactions that seem to occur between collagen and the L-iduronate residues in the proteoglycan.

Heparin is classified together with other glycosaminoglycans, although it is not a connective-tissue polysaccharide. It is stored in mast cells located beneath the endothelium of most blood vessels. Heparin has two well-established biological properties:

(1) It acts as a blood anticoagulant. Heparin is the most acidic of all the glycosamino-glycans and interferes with blood clotting by binding to several of the proteins required for the process. It has been used clinically for many years as a blood anticoagulant.

(2) It activates lipoprotein lipase. This is a lipase found in muscle and adipose tissue which hydrolyses triglycerides of lipoproteins, and is particularly important in "clearing" lipoprotein-bound triglycerides from the blood after digestion of a fatty meal.

Synthesis and breakdown of glycosaminoglycans

The glycosaminoglycans are synthesized as their protein complexes in the internal membrane systems of the cell, and are then secreted in a completed form (figure 8.11). Several different phases can be recognized in the synthetic process:

(1) Synthesis of protein.
(2) Addition of monosaccharide units from nucleoside diphosphate sugars.
(3) Further modification, e.g. sulphation.
(4) Secretion.

The formation of the protein component occurs on ribosomes attached to the membranes of the rough endoplasmic reticulum and the newly synthesized polypeptide chains are translocated to the cisternal side of the membrane. The molecules then pass through the cisternae of the endoplasmic reticulum and to the membrane system of the Golgi apparatus. During this period, the carbohydrate chains are built up by addition of one monosaccharide at a time from the appropriate nucleoside diphosphate sugar precursors. These reactions require the presence of a series of specific glycosyltransferases which occur as part of the membrane system or are located within the cisternae. The transferases are highly specific for the donor nucleoside diphosphate sugar, the acceptor molecule and for the type of linkage synthesized, including its anomeric configuration. This high specificity ensures that the polymer is produced with a reproducible sequence of monosaccharides linked together in a reproducible manner.

Figure 8.12 shows the series of enzymic reactions leading to the synthesis of chondroitin sulphate. This requires the coordination of different enzymes, all of which work in a specific sequence dictated by their acceptor specificity. None can add glycosyl units out of turn because of this specificity and, as the molecule is built up one unit at a time, its acceptor structure changes from that recognized by one enzyme to that for the next in sequence. The enzymes may recognize parts of the acceptor beyond the terminal residue. Thus enzyme 3 will add galactose to an

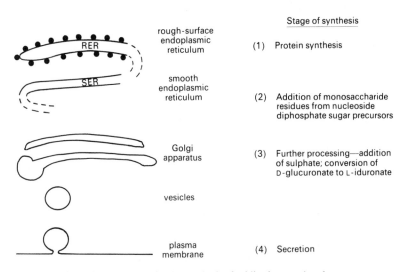

Stage of synthesis

rough-surface
endoplasmic
reticulum   (1)   Protein synthesis

smooth
endoplasmic
reticulum   (2)   Addition of monosaccharide
                           residues from nucleoside
                           diphosphate sugar precursors

Golgi
apparatus   (3)   Further processing—addition
                           of sulphate; conversion of
                           D-glucuronate to L-iduronate

vesicles

plasma
membrane   (4)   Secretion

Figure 8.11   Scheme for the synthesis of acidic glycosaminoglycans.

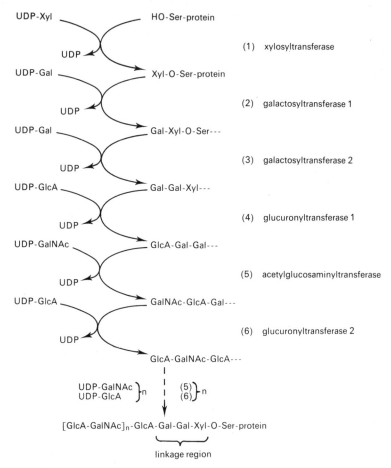

Figure 8.12 Sequence of transferases involved in the synthesis of chondroitin sulphate.
n = approximately 50.

acceptor with the sequence Gal-Xyl-Ser-protein but will not recognize
the sequence Gal-Gal-Xyl-Ser-protein as a suitable substrate. After the
linkage region has been completed, chain extension occurs by repeated
alternating action of enzymes 5 and 6 to synthesize the full-length
polymer.

Further modification may take place after completion of the polysaccharide chain. It is at this stage that sulphate groups are added by
transfer from the coenzyme phosphoadenosine phosphosulphate. In

heparin (which contains N-sulphate groups, table 8.4) the amino sugars are first incorporated into the polymer as their N-acetyl derivatives, but then the N-acetyl groups are removed by hydrolysis and replaced by sulphate. In the case of glycosaminoglycans which contain L-iduronate as a residue, the polymer is first synthesized as a D-glucuronate derivative, and then the necessary epimerization at C-5 to give L-iduronate takes place in the polymer. This is an unusual reaction in that epimerization of sugars more often occurs with the sugars as their phosphate or nucleoside diphosphate derivatives (chapter 3). Not all of the D-glucuronate residues become modified, so that L-iduronate-containing glycosaminoglycans usually contain a proportion of unmodified D-glucuronate residues.

The glycosaminoglycans of connective tissues undergo continual turnover such that the average life of an individual polymer molecule is only a few days. During breakdown, the proteoglycan complexes are first attacked by proteolytic enzymes, and the freed glycosaminoglycans are taken up by cells (either locally or via the circulation to the liver). Once in the cell, they are taken up by lysosomes where the main process of hydrolysis occurs. In certain congenital human diseases, one or other of the hydrolytic lysosomal enzymes is missing. When this occurs, there is usually a massive accumulation of undegraded or partly degraded glycosaminoglycans in the lysosomes of many tissues, and glycosaminoglycans also appear in the urine. Such diseases affect the degradation of dermatan sulphate and heparan sulphate in particular (both of which contain L-iduronate), and in some of these cases lysosomal iduronidase is absent.

Breakdown of the proteoglycans of articular cartilage is also involved in the development of rheumatoid arthritis. (The articular cartilage covers the ends of bones in joints.) Lysosomal enzymes are released into the articular cartilage in abnormally large amounts, and this causes erosion of the matrix, so that friction develops and the joint is unable to move smoothly.

CHAPTER NINE

COMPLEX CARBOHYDRATE POLYMERS

The glycoproteins and glycolipids are considered together as complex carbohydrate polymers. Such compounds typically contain oligosaccharide chains covalently attached to either protein or lipid. The oligosaccharide structures are frequently complex and may be made up of several different types of sugar residue.

Complex carbohydrates are usually, but not always, found outside cells, where they occur as part of the outer surface of the cell or are soluble components of extracellular fluids such as blood. Several different functions have been suggested for complex carbohydrates, and these are of two general types. One type of function seems to depend on the general physical properties of the molecules, for example, the glycoprotein mucins which lubricate and protect epithelial surfaces fall into this category. Other functions depend more on the exact structure of the carbohydrate chains which provide specific recognition sites required for antigen-antibody, hormone-receptor, and cell-cell interactions.

Glycoproteins

General structure

The term *glycoprotein* covers a wide range of compounds of diverse structures. They all have a protein chain to which is covalently linked one or more carbohydrate chains. In its widest sense, the term *glycoprotein* also covers polymers such as bacterial cell-wall peptidoglycan and the protein-linked acidic glycosaminoglycans (see chapter 8).

The proportion of carbohydrate in different glycoproteins ranges from

Table 9.1 Characteristic monosaccharide components of glycoproteins

Monosaccharide	Abbreviation	Biosynthetic precursor
D-galactose	Gal	UDP-Gal
D-mannose	Man	GDP-Man
L-fucose (6-deoxy-L-galactose)	Fuc	GDP-Fuc
N-acetylglucosamine	GlcNAc	UDP-GlcNAc
N-acetylgalactosamine	GalNAc	UDP-GalNAc
sialic acids, e.g.		
N-acetylneuraminic acid	NeuNAc	CMP-NeuNAc
N-glycolylneuraminic acid	NeuNGl	CMP-NeuNGl
glucose (collagen only)	Glc	UDP-Glc
D-xylose (plants)	Xyl	UDP-Xyl
L-arabinose (plants)	Ara	UDP-Ara

small (2–3 % of the total weight) to large (up to 90 % in some epithelial mucins). In some there is only one oligosaccharide chain for each peptide chain, whereas in others many oligosaccharides are joined to the same peptide. The carbohydrate component may be very simple (one monosaccharide residue) or complex with perhaps fifteen monosaccharides of several different types. Table 9.1 lists the monosaccharides most commonly found in glycoproteins.

Unlike the glycosaminoglycans (chapter 8), the glycoproteins do not have simple repeating units and do not have uronic acids. However, some are acidic in character and the charged groups of these glycoproteins are due to the presence of one of a group of compounds known as the *sialic acids*. These are derivatives of a nine-carbon sugar, neuraminic acid, which contains both a carboxylate group and an amino group, with the latter most commonly substituted with an acetyl group or a glycolyl group. The structure of N-acetylneuraminic acid is shown in figure 1.8 (p. 13). When present in glycoproteins, the sialic acids are usually found at the non-reducing terminal ends of the carbohydrate chains, that is, at the exposed outer ends. Figure 9.1 shows the structures of some typical glycoproteins.

Only a few different types of linkages are used to join the carbohydrate to the peptide chain in the glycoproteins. The four most common types are:

(1) An N-glycosidic linkage between N-acetylglucosamine and the amide nitrogen of an asparagine residue of the protein. This type of linkage is of wide occurrence and has been found in a number of animal and plant glycoproteins.
(2) An O-glycosidic linkage between N-acetylgalactosamine and the hydroxyl group of a serine or threonine residue in the protein. This type is found in animal glycoproteins such as the mucins and blood group substances.

(3) An O-glycosidic linkage between galactose and a hydroxylysine residue of the protein. This type is found in collagen.

(4) An O-glycosidic linkage between L-arabinose and a hydroxyproline residue of the protein. This is found in the extensin of plant cell walls.

All of these linkages are glycosidic, and it is significant that during glycoprotein synthesis (p. 155) the peptide is synthesized first and the carbohydrates are added afterwards. In contrast, the linkage between carbohydrate and peptide in bacterial peptidoglycan (p. 135) is an amide bond between the carboxylate group of the carbohydrate and the amino group of an amino acid. In peptidoglycan synthesis, the amino acids are added to the carbohydrate, so the different type of linkage can be ascribed to the different order of assembly of the molecules during synthesis.

(1)   Pig submandibular gland glycoprotein (salivary mucin)

$$GalNAc\alpha(1 \rightarrow 3)Gal\beta(1 \rightarrow 3)GalNAc\beta\text{-}O\text{-}Ser\text{-}protein$$
$$\begin{array}{cc} 2 & 6 \\ \uparrow & \uparrow \\ Fuc\alpha1 & NeuNAc\alpha2 \end{array}$$

(2)   Human immunoglobulin G

$$GlcNAc\beta(1 \rightarrow 2)Man\alpha$$
$$\begin{array}{c} 1 \\ \downarrow \\ 6 \end{array}$$
$$NeuNAc\alpha(1 \rightarrow 2)Gal\beta(1 \rightarrow 6)GlcNAc\beta(1 \rightarrow 2)Man\alpha(1 \rightarrow 3)Man\alpha(1 \rightarrow 3)GlcNAc\beta\text{-}N\text{-}Asn\text{-}protein$$
$$\begin{array}{c} 4 \\ \uparrow \\ 1 \\ Fuc\alpha(1 \rightarrow 3)GlcNAc\beta \end{array}$$

(3)   Bromelain (pineapple stem protease)

$$Man\alpha(1 \rightarrow 2)Man\alpha$$
$$\begin{array}{c} 1 \\ \downarrow \\ 2 \end{array}$$
$$Fuc\alpha(1 \rightarrow 6)Man\alpha$$
$$\begin{array}{c} 1 \\ \downarrow \\ 3 \end{array}$$
$$Xyl\beta(1 \rightarrow 4)GlcNAc\beta(1 \rightarrow 4)GlcNAc\beta\text{-}N\text{-}Asn\text{-}protein$$

(4)   Extensin (plant cell wall)

Gal-Ara-O-hydroxyproline-protein

Figure 9.1   Examples of some oligosaccharide structures of glycoproteins.

Soluble and membrane-bound glycoproteins

Many of the proteins found in extracellular fluids such as blood are glycoproteins. These are soluble in water and any amino acids they may have with hydrophobic groups are usually buried inside the molecule. The presence of carbohydrate tends to make such glycoproteins more water-soluble because of the hydrophilic character of the carbohydrate.

In contrast, membrane-bound glycoproteins form part of the membrane structure and therefore have to interact with the lipid of the membrane. Membrane glycoproteins have been found to have one or more regions of the peptide sequence in which hydrophobic amino acids predominate, and such regions are believed to associate with the lipid layer of the membrane. The carbohydrate component of plasma membrane glycoproteins is present on that part of the molecule which is on the outside of the cell, and rarely or never occurs on other parts of the molecule. Although the carbohydrate content of plasma membranes is relatively small (about 5% in red blood cells, less in some cell types), it is nevertheless important because it is present on the outer surface of the cell where interactions with the environment take place. Glycoproteins are also found on some intracellular membranes such as those of the mitochondria, lysosomes, nucleus and sarcoplasmic reticulum.

One plasma membrane glycoprotein which has been studied in some detail is the major glycoprotein ("glycophorin") of red blood cells. The amino-acid sequence shows a hydrophilic region at the C-terminal end, a central hydrophobic region, and a second hydrophilic region at the N-terminal end (figure 9.2). The carbohydrate is confined solely to the N-terminal region. It is likely that the glycophorin is organized in the membrane such that the hydrophobic region is in the lipid bilayer and the two hydrophilic regions project either side with the carbohydrate-containing N-terminal end on the outer face. This general arrangement may occur in other membrane glycoproteins. In larger glycoproteins, the molecules may have several hydrophobic regions and may traverse the membrane several times.

Synthesis

The sequence of events leading to the biosynthesis of glycoproteins resembles that described for the acidic glycosaminoglycans (p. 148). The protein is synthesized first on the membrane-bound ribosomes of the rough endoplasmic reticulum, and is then glycosylated during passage

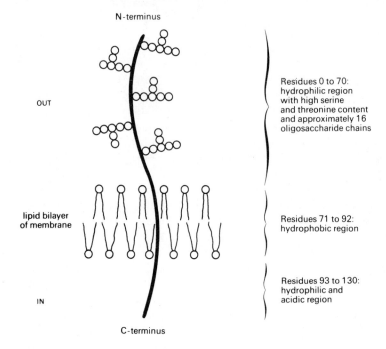

N-terminus

OUT

Residues 0 to 70:
hydrophilic region
with high serine
and threonine content
and approximately 16
oligosaccharide chains

lipid bilayer
of membrane

Residues 71 to 92:
hydrophobic region

Residues 93 to 130:
hydrophilic and
acidic region

IN

C-terminus

Figure 9.2   Glycophorin—the major glycoprotein of the red-cell membrane.

through the endoplasmic reticulum and Golgi apparatus. In the case of soluble glycoproteins, the product is released from the secretory vesicle when this fuses with the plasma membrane. For cell-surface glycoproteins, the product is already part of the vesicle membrane (probably by virtue of a hydrophobic peptide region) and is retained by the plasma membrane when fusion takes place (figure 9.3).

It has been found that a number of membrane and secretory proteins are first synthesized with an extra length of peptide present at the N-terminal end (the end which is first synthesized). These "signal peptides" are between 15 and 30 amino acids long and are mainly hydrophobic. They are believed to initiate attachment of the growing protein chain, together with ribosome and messenger RNA, to the membrane of the rough endoplasmic reticulum. They may allow the cell to distinguish between "export" proteins and those designed to stay within the cell which are synthesized on free ribosomes. During synthesis, the growing protein is transferred into the cisternae of the endoplasmic reticulum, and the signal peptide is removed by hydrolysis during further processing of the molecule.

Two rather different mechanisms exist for addition of the mono-saccharide residues during glycoprotein synthesis. For the glycoproteins containing O-glycosidic linkages (to serine, threonine or hydroxylysine), the monosaccharides are added one at a time from nucleoside diphos-phate sugar precursors in reactions catalysed by glycosyltransferases. Such glycosyltransferases are specific both for the acceptor and for the

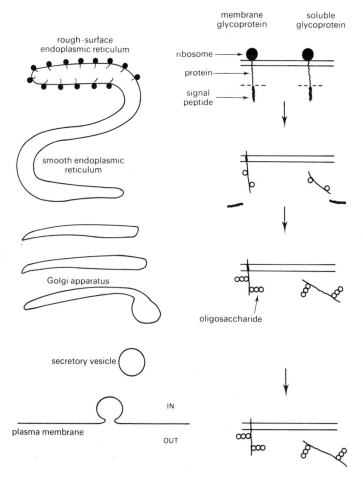

Figure 9.3 Synthesis of soluble and membrane-bound glycoproteins in the internal membrane systems of the cell.

sugar and nucleotide components of the nucleoside ·diphosphate sugar donor. This is essentially the same mechanism as that described for the acidic glycosaminoglycans (p. 149), which also contain O-glycosidic linkages between carbohydrate and protein. However, for glycoproteins in which carbohydrate is attached to protein via an N-glycosidic linkage to asparagine, a rather different mechanism operates which involves a lipid carrier present in the internal membrane system of the cell. This carrier is a polyisoprenol phosphate derivative, and thus resembles the carrier involved in synthesis of bacterial peptidoglycan (p. 135). However, in mammals (and probably in many other eukaryotic cells, including yeast and higher plants) the polyisoprenol is one of a family of lipids with 80 to 100 carbon atoms in the chain known as the *dolichols*. Retinol may also act as lipid carrier in some systems.

During the synthesis of such glycoproteins, an oligosaccharide chain is first built up as a dolichol diphosphate derivative, and is then transferred as a unit to the protein. Further modification then takes place—some carbohydrate residues are removed, and then other residues are added by direct transfer from nucleoside diphosphate sugars.

For the direct transfer mechanism of glycoprotein synthesis, it is assumed that the glycosyltransfer reactions take place within the cisternae of the endoplasmic reticulum and Golgi apparatus, and that therefore the nucleoside diphosphate sugars must pass across the membranes from the cytosol where they are synthesized. It is also likely that the nucleotide products (e.g. UDP or perhaps UMP after hydrolysis of UDP) must pass back into the cytosol. Specific transport mechanisms are therefore assumed to exist in the membranes. For the indirect transfer mechanism involving dolichol phosphate intermediates, it is less clear that transport of the nucleotides is required. This could take place by assembly of the oligosaccharides on the cytosol face of the membrane, followed by transport through the membrane on the carrier (as proposed for synthesis of bacterial peptidoglycan).

Much of what is known about the synthesis of glycoproteins is based on studies of mammalian systems. However, the available evidence suggests that similar mechanisms exist in other eukaryotic cells.

Glycolipids

Glycolipids are compounds in which carbohydrate is linked glycosidically to a lipid to produce a derivative which has both hydrophobic and hydrophilic regions. Glycolipids are common components of membranes, where the hydrophobic region is buried in the other lipids of the membrane, and the carbohydrate extends into the aqueous phase. Although glycolipids are present in most plasma membranes, they are found in particularly high concentrations in the central nervous system of animals.

The structures of some glycolipids are shown in figure 9.4. The glycolipids of mammalian cells are mainly glycosphingolipids in which the number of sugar residues may be one or more. The oligosaccharide components of glycolipids often bear a striking resemblance to those of glycoproteins produced within the same tissue. When these structures are compared, it is found that the "core" region linking the carbohydrate to protein or lipid differs between glycoprotein and glycolipid, but that the external parts of the chains are identical. Thus the external sequences of the soluble blood group substance glycoproteins are identical to those of the glycolipids found on the surface of red blood cells. Such substances have identical antigenic specificities (p. 163) because it is these external sequences which are recognized by antibody molecules.

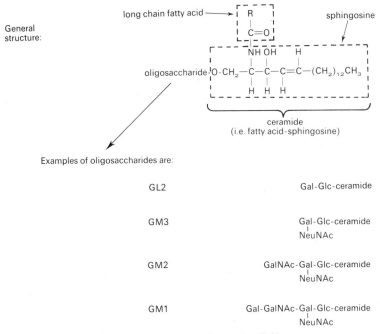

Figure 9.4   Structures of some glycolipids.

Disorders of complex carbohydrate metabolism

In certain rare inherited diseases, one or other of the enzymes involved in the metabolism of complex carbohydrates is absent (or present in an inactive form). Such genetic defects could affect either the synthetic or the degradative enzymes of complex carbohydrate metabolism. However, defects in synthetic enzymes are not usually seen clinically because, if the compound affected is essential to life, the foetus does not survive to birth. Defects in degradative enzymes usually have a more delayed effect. Glycoproteins and glycolipids undergo continual turnover, as do most components of living organisms. Their breakdown generally depends upon uptake into lysosomes, with subsequent hydrolysis by specific hydrolytic enzymes. If one of these enzymes is absent, then glycolipids and sometimes glycoproteins accumulate in the lysosomes. This is a gradual process and may take several years to become apparent. Eventually the lysosomes become excessively swollen with undegraded materials and become mechanically damaged, thus releasing proteolytic enzymes (cathepsins) into the cell.

One example of such a genetic defect is seen in Tay-Sachs disease, in which there is an excessive accumulation of the ganglioside GM2 (for structure see figure 9.4). This occurs because the enzyme which hydrolyses the terminal *N*-acetylgalactosamine of GM2 (to convert it to GM3) is lacking in individuals with this disease.

Functions of complex carbohydrates

Complex carbohydrates have a range of different biological functions (table 9.2). Sometimes there is a clear relationship between the carbohydrate content of the polymer and its biological role, but in other cases the function of the carbohydrate moiety is not well established.

The mucins are a group of glycoproteins in mucous secretions of epithelia in the digestive, urinogenital and other tracts of animals. They have a high molecular weight and high carbohydrate content, and usually bear charged sialic acid groups. This structure gives them a high viscosity in solution, in rather a similar way to the glycosaminoglycans (chapter 8). Their function is to lubricate and protect the epithelia. The protective role is partly a physical one—the viscous solutions form a thick tenacious layer which covers the epithelia and protects them from abrasive damage. For the digestive tract, it has also been suggested that the mucins could protect the epithelia from digestion by proteolytic enzymes present in

Table 9.2   Functions of complex carbohydrates

Function	Examples
structural	collagen
lubrication and protection	epithelial mucins, synovial fluid glycoprotein
transport	caeruloplasmin (copper carrier), transferrin (iron carrier)
food reserve	seed glycoproteins, egg white ovalbumin, milk casein
hormone	thyroglobulin, interstitial cell stimulating hormone
enzyme	glucose oxidase, invertase, RNase B, bromelain
antifreeze	blood glycoproteins of Antarctic fish
receptors	cell surface receptors for insulin, acetylcholine, luteinizing hormone, cholera toxin
cell recognition and adhesion	lectins, LETS glycoprotein
antigens	blood group substances, bacterial cell-wall components
antibodies	mammalian immunoglobulins
others	rhodopsin, blood clotting factors, ricin (a plant toxin)

digestive fluids. According to this, the large protease molecules would be excluded from the surface region by a network of glycoprotein molecules, and yet the small products of digestion could pass through the network and be absorbed by the epithelia. The mucins themselves are slowly degraded by the enzymes and also the low pH of the stomach, but are replaced by continual synthesis, so that the epithelia are always protected.

Many extracellular proteins contain at least a small amount of covalently-bound carbohydrate. The function of the carbohydrate in such molecules is not always known. Thus, for enzymes, the catalytic activity is not usually affected, whether the carbohydrate is present or not, and carbohydrates never seem to be involved in the active site of the enzyme. However, in some glycoprotein enzymes, the carbohydrate may help to stabilize the molecules and thus increase their biological life. Yeast produces invertase in a series of isoenzymes which differ from each other only in the amount of carbohydrate (mannose) present. These enzymes all have similar catalytic activities, but the greater the carbohydrate content, the more stable is the enzyme to denaturation.

An unusual group of glycoproteins has been found in the blood of certain antarctic fish. These have the ability to depress the freezing-point of solutions by an anomalously large amount. On a weight basis, they are better freezing-point depressants than sodium chloride. The reason for this anomalous behaviour may be related to their highly hydrated and expanded structure which could interfere with the formation of ice crystals.

Specific interactions of complex carbohydrates

Glycoproteins and glycolipids participate in a number of specific binding reactions in which carbohydrate sequences are recognized by complementary sites on proteins. Such reactions can involve both soluble molecules and those present on cell surfaces, and are important in antigen-antibody reactions, hormone receptors and cell–cell interactions.

Antigenic carbohydrates

The antigen-antibody reaction is one in which a normally foreign compound—the antigen—reacts with an antibody produced by an animal. Such reactions are non-covalent but are usually very specific. A wide range of different antibodies is present in mammalian blood, each antibody being specific for a particular antigen. The antibody recognizes one particular region on the antigen molecule which is known as the *antigenic determinant*. There is considerable interest in antigen-antibody reactions, both for their medical importance and because the antibodies are extremely useful tools for the specific detection and measurement of proteins.

Antigens may be proteins, glycoproteins or in some cases glycolipids. Although proteins lacking carbohydrate can be antigenic, where carbohydrate is present this is frequently the antigenic determinant on the molecule. This is perhaps because the carbohydrate is typically present at the surface of the molecule, and is therefore most accessible to the antibody. Antigens are also present on cell surfaces and, here again, the determinants are often carbohydrates if only because the outermost surface of cells is characterized by its carbohydrate.

Table 9.3 Blood groups of the ABO system in man. Agglutination occurs when cells of one blood group are mixed with plasma containing antibody to the antigenic determinant of that group

Blood type	Oligosaccharide type on red cells	Antibody in serum	Types of serum which cause agglutination of cells
O	H substance	anti-A, anti-B	none
A	A substance	anti-B	O, B
B	B substance	anti-A	O, A
AB	A and B substances	none	O, A, B

Except in certain pathological conditions, antibodies are not developed against normal components of the animal's own blood and tissues. However, cells of other types are recognized as being foreign by the animal's immune system. A well-known example of such behaviour is seen in the reactions of red blood cells in man. Landsteiner in 1900 first described the ABO system of blood grouping according to the reactions of red cells with the serum of other individuals (table 9.3). Introduction of the "wrong" type of cell into serum (e.g. cells of type A into serum of type B) causes the cells to clump together ("agglutinate") because the red cell antigens react with antibodies present in the serum. Since antibodies have multiple binding sites, when one site reacts with one cell and another site with a second cell, the two cells become linked. In the presence of larger numbers of antibody molecules, large clumps of cells are formed.

The antigenic determinants on the red cell surface which are responsible for the ABO grouping are carbohydrates (mainly glycolipids but also perhaps glycoproteins) which have oligosaccharide side-chains characteristic of their particular blood group. The amounts of such antigens in red cells are rather small, which makes it difficult to determine their chemical structure. However, complex carbohydrates with the same oligosaccharide composition as the red-cell antigens are often found in soluble form in body fluids of the same individual. In particular, the fluid produced in ovarian cysts is a rich source of blood group specific glycoproteins. These compounds have been very useful experimentally, because they can be isolated in large amounts and their detailed structure determined.

Figure 9.5 shows the relationship between the structure of the blood group substances and their antigenic behaviour. The H substance produced by individuals of blood group O is not an antigen in humans but, if injected into other animals such as cows, will provoke an immune response there.

The blood group substances can be interconverted experimentally. Thus an α-galactosidase converts human B cells into type O cells by removing the terminal galactose from B-substance to give H-substance. Similarly, type O cells can be converted to type A or B cells by incubation with the appropriate glycosyltransferase and the UDP derivative of N-acetylgalactosamine or galactose respectively.

Blood groups are inherited from parents according to classical Mendelian mechanisms. The glycosyltransferases for the synthesis of complex carbohydrates are coded for by particular genes, and the complement of genes possessed by an individual determines the type of

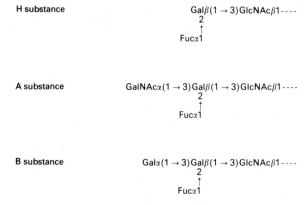

Figure 9.5 Structures of the oligosaccharide antigenic determinants of blood group substances.

oligosaccharide chains synthesized. Most humans have the necessary enzymes to synthesize H-substance, but some lack enzymes for further modification of this structure. These are individuals of blood group O. Other individuals have either a glycosyltransferase for adding *N*-acetyl-galactosamine in an $\alpha(1 \rightarrow 3)$ linkage to the galactose residue of H-substance (type A), or for adding galactose linked in the same way (type B). Others have both of these enzymes and synthesize a mixture of blood group substances (type AB).

Although this relationship between glycoprotein structure and anti-genic behaviour was worked out from studies on soluble glycoproteins, it is now clear that the characteristic blood group oligosaccharide chains are synthesized by many different cells in the body. The antigenic deter-minants characteristic of the individual are found in glycoproteins of body fluids such as saliva or milk, and in glycoproteins and glycolipids of many different cell types.

Since the discovery of the ABO system of blood grouping, some 160 different human antigens have been found on the red cells, although many of these occur only rarely. The chemical structures of many of the determinants of these antigens is still not known, but for at least some of them a carbohydrate oligosaccharide has been implicated. Thus the determinants for the M and N antigens are located on the major glycoprotein (glycophorin) of the red-cell membrane. The difference between the M and N antigens seems to be that the M antigen has one more sialic-acid group than the N antigen.

Cell surface receptors

The outer surface of the plasma membrane of cells contains a variety of specific receptors by which hormones and other agents can interact with the cell and provoke a physiological response. Different cell types have different combinations of receptors, and the ability of a cell to respond to a particular hormone often depends on whether or not the appropriate receptor is present on the membrane. In addition to hormone receptors, other specific receptors in cells include those for transmitter substances in nerve cells, for antigens in fibroblasts, and for toxins in many cell types. In a number of cases there is evidence that such receptors depend on their detailed carbohydrate structure for specific interactions, but only in a few cases has the role of carbohydrate been established with little doubt. One well-established example is that of the receptor to cholera toxin, and this can be regarded as a useful model system which is analogous to certain hormone-receptor interactions.

Cholera toxin is secreted by the pathogenic bacterium *Vibrio cholerae* and its main effect is to cause excessive secretion of water and salts into the intestine, so that the tissues of the infected patient become dehydrated. If this effect is not controlled, the loss of water from the body becomes lethal.

Cholera toxin is a protein consisting of a single type-A subunit surrounded by a ring of five type-B subunits. The toxin binds to target cells by interaction with the ganglioside GM1 which is the receptor on the cell surface. The binding leads to a conformational change in the membrane, such that part of the A subunit of the toxin is separated from the rest of the toxin and enters the cell. The internalized fragment catalyses a transfer of ADP-ribose from NAD onto the regulatory nucleotide binding protein of the adenylate cyclase:

$$NAD + \text{regulator protein} \rightarrow \text{ADP-ribose-regulator protein} + \text{nicotinamide}$$

The effect of ADP-ribosylation is to inhibit the normal GTPase turn-off mechanism of the adenylate cyclase (p. 172) so the adenylate cyclase is fixed in the fully active form. Consequently the cyclic AMP level in the cell is considerably elevated. In fact, cholera toxin has the effect of elevating cyclic AMP levels in many cell types but, in the diseased state, the principal cells affected are the secretory cells of the intestine. Such cells respond to elevated cyclic AMP levels by drastically increasing the rate of secretion of electrolytes and fluid.

A group of mammalian hormones (thyrotropin, luteinizing hormone, human chorionic gonadotropin, and follicle-stimulating hormone) are closely related to each other, and their mechanism of interaction with the cell surface resembles that of cholera toxin. All four hormones have two types of subunits (α and β) of which the α-subunit is common to all the hormones, and exerts its effect by activating adenylate cyclase. The β-subunits of the hormones are different from each other (although they have some amino-acid sequences in common with each other) and it is these which bind to their own receptors. It is suggested that binding provokes a conformational change in the hormone, as a result of which the α-subunit is either translocated into or through the membrane to activate the adenylate cyclase. The β-subunit therefore specifies the particular hormone activity to be expressed by the nature of the receptors it binds to.

Another type of specific interaction is involved in the mechanism of removal of certain glycoproteins from the blood of mammals. Blood glycoproteins undergo continual turnover: they are synthesized, released into the blood, and then eventually (after a period characteristic for the particular protein) they are taken up by other cells to be hydrolysed in the lysosomes. One example of such a glycoprotein is the copper-carrying protein,.caeruloplasmin. The native glycoprotein has carbohydrate chains with sialic acid at the non-reducing end, joined to a galactose residue at the penultimate position. If caeruloplasmin is isolated, made radioactive, and injected into a test rabbit, it persists in the circulation with an average life of about 56 hours. However, if such caeruloplasmin is first treated with sialidase (to remove the terminal sialic acid residues) and is then injected into a test animal, it is removed from the circulation in about 10 minutes (Ashwell & Morell). The recognition site on the modified caeruloplasmin seems to be the newly exposed galactose residue, since further modification either by oxidation with galactose oxidase, or by "covering" the galactose with sialic acid, decreases its rate of removal.

Further experiments showed that the desialylated protein is removed by liver cells (hepatocytes) which have a specific cell surface glycoprotein capable of binding to the modified caeruloplasmin. Binding of the protein is followed by its uptake into the lysosomes of the cells where it is hydrolysed.

These findings have been extended to other circulating glycoproteins. In a number of these, their continued survival in the circulation depends on the presence of a terminal sialic-acid residue, and exposure of a penultimate galactose residue provides a recognition site for the hepatocyte receptor. It is possible that *in vivo* ageing of such glycoproteins may take place such that the rather labile sialic-acid residues are gradually lost until sufficient galactose residues are exposed for the glycoprotein to be recognized by the liver.

Cell–cell interactions

The complex carbohydrates on the surfaces of cells play an important role in communication and interaction between cells. Cells within a tissue interact with each other so that adhesion, growth, differentiation and size are all controlled in a coordinated manner. If this system of communication is disrupted, the cells may grow in a less controlled manner characteristic of cancer cells.

The molecular mechanisms which control the differentiation of many tissues are not known in detail because of the difficulty of designing suitable experiments to study them. However, there are some systems which lend themselves more readily to experimental manipulation, and these will be considered here as models which may have wider implications for cell–cell interactions in general. Such experiments have been carried out using blood cells, cells grown in tissue culture, and primitive organisms such as sponges and slime moulds.

Human red blood cells have an average life of about 120 days in the circulation, and gradually age during this time. Old cells are taken up by the Kupffer cells of the liver and are phagocytized. This process involves specific recognition of the old red cells (as distinct from young cells) by the Kupffer cells, and so is an example of specific cell–cell interaction. When young red blood cells are experimentally treated with sialidase to remove the external sialic-acid residues, and are then injected into test animals, they are removed from the circulation very quickly. This suggests that the Kupffer cells recognize desialylated carbohydrate structures on the surface of the cells. It has been proposed that, during normal ageing, the red cells lose sialic-acid residues until sufficient new residues are exposed on the surface to allow them to be recognized as old cells by receptors on the Kupffer cells. This type of interaction resembles that occurring in the removal of desialylated plasma glycoproteins by the liver (p. 166), although in that case different cells, the hepatocytes, are involved in uptake.

The slime moulds have been used to study the development and differentiation of cells at a relatively simple level. In the presence of a plentiful supply of food (bacteria), the slime moulds exist as a population of separate and identical amoeboid cells which feed on the bacteria, grow and divide. When the food runs out, the cells start to associate together and become cohesive until a multicellular "slug" is formed of large numbers (up to 100 000) of similar cells. Cells in different parts of the slug then start to differentiate to form a fruiting body in which some cells form a stalk and other cells produce spores which can survive unfavourable conditions until food again becomes available.

During the first part of this process, the cells change from the non-cohesive amoeboid type to a cohesive type. It has been found that the cohesive cells have two surface proteins not present in the non-cohesive cells, and that these proteins are "lectins" (p. 169) capable of recognizing and binding to a specific carbohydrate group (probably galactose) on the surface of adjacent cells. If the synthesis of one of these proteins is blocked by mutation, the cells are no longer able to associate together. In these organisms there appears to be a clear relationship between the presence of a lectin-carbohydrate interaction on the cell surface and the ability of the cells to associate together to form a simple multicellular organism.

Another simple cell-association system occurs with certain marine sponges which can be dissociated into separate cells by squeezing them through a fine-mesh cloth. The separated cells will then aggregate together again in a process which is species-specific. As long ago as 1907, Wilson mixed together cells from red and yellow sponges and found that the cells sorted themselves such that those of the red species associated together into groups and those from the yellow species associated into different groups.

A factor required for aggregation has been isolated from the sponge *Microciones parthena*. It is a large protein-polysaccharide complex which contains uronic-acid residues. A second component present on the surface of the cells will bind to this aggregation factor, and separate cells can become linked together indirectly via the aggregation factor. The second component on the cell surface can be released by osmotic shock, and cells treated in this way are no longer able to aggregate.

Many different types of cells can now be grown in tissue culture. When cultured cells are grown on a surface such as that of a Petri dish, they grow and divide until the whole surface of the plate is covered with a single layer of cells. Further growth then usually stops, due to what is known as "contact inhibition" of growth, which occurs when each cell is in contact with other cells surrounding it. However, cultured cells can be modified or "transformed" by treatment with certain viruses or with carcinogenic chemicals. (Transformed cells have properties in common with cancer cells, and have been studied extensively because of this). Transformed cells often do not show the contact inhibition response of the parent strain, and continue to grow beyond a monolayer to form cultures several layers thick. It seems that in normal cells there is a restriction on growth which depends on cell–cell interaction, but that in transformed cells there is no such check on growth. Malignant cancer cells grown in culture can show similar growth characteristics to those of the transformed cells.

The surface carbohydrates of transformed cells have been compared with those of the parent strains. In some there is a significant difference between the two cell types: the transformed cells have carbohydrates with a rather different structure from the parent cells. Thus in control hamster kidney cells, the ganglioside GM3 predominates, but in transformed cells GM3 is decreased to a quarter of the control value, and the ganglioside GL2 (figure 9.4), which is a precursor of GM3, is present instead.

For other cultured cells, changes occur in the glycoprotein composition after transformation with viruses or chemicals. Thus fibroblasts and myoblasts have a surface glycoprotein known as LETS ("large external transformation-sensitive glycoprotein", also known as "fibronectin") on their surface, whereas transformed cells usually have either no LETS or reduced amounts of it. Purified LETS added to cultures of transformed cells induces increased attachment of cells and causes them to align together like normal cells. It has therefore been suggested that LETS plays a role in the adhesion of cells and in controlling their normal growth. The tumorogenicity (capacity to form tumours after injection into test animals) of cells is generally greater in cells with small amounts of LETS.

In 1970, Roseman proposed that some interactions between cells could take place by glycosyltransferases present on the cell surface. According to this hypothesis, the glycosyltransferases bind to their normal substrates (oligosaccharide side-chains of glycoproteins or glycolipids) on the surfaces of adjacent cells and thus join the cells together. As an extension of this proposal, cell separation could take place if the second substrate (a nucleoside diphosphate sugar) of the enzyme became available to permit completion of the glycosyltransferase reaction with subsequent separation of the enzyme and product. As yet there is no conclusive evidence to support this interesting idea.

Lectins

The term *lectin* is used to describe proteins which bind carbohydrates specifically but non-covalently. Although lectins were originally found in plant seeds, they are now known to occur more widely, and have been

Table 9.4 Lectins

Origin	Carbohydrate group bound	Blood group
Lima bean	GalNAc	A
Lotus	α-Fuc	H
Jack bean (concanavalin A)	α-Man, α-Glc	
Wheat germ	(GlcNAc)$_2$	
Horseshoe crab	sialic acid	
Sea snail	sialic acid	
Peanut	Gal	

reported in fungi, bacteria, lichens, snails, fish and mammals. Table 9.4 lists some examples of lectins.

Lectins are of particular interest as experimental tools to detect specific carbohydrate groups and for purification of carbohydrate-containing compounds. Some lectins have the property of agglutinating human red-blood cells, and can be used in typing blood and for studying the structure of blood group substances.

The biological functions of lectins are not always known, but some may be involved in carbohydrate transport, in specific recognition, in cohesion or in antibody-like binding of carbohydrates. It is possible that some bind carbohydrate by some chance configuration complementary to that of the carbohydrate, and that their true function lies elsewhere. Some lectins have been described earlier. Liver hepatocytes have a lectin which binds glycoproteins with exposed terminal galactose residues (p. 166) and slime moulds synthesize a lectin for binding to receptors on cell surfaces during aggregation (p. 168). Antibodies which react with carbohydrate determinants can be regarded as a special form of lectin. Many, but not all, lectins are glycoproteins.

CHAPTER TEN

HORMONAL REGULATION

The individual cells of multicellular organisms are regulated by centralized control systems so that their response to physiological stimuli can be coordinated together. The two main methods of achieving this coordination are through the nervous system and by chemical control through hormones. In all but the simplest animals, hormones are secreted by specialized endocrine glands, and are carried in the blood to their target tissues.

There are several different aspects to the understanding of hormonal regulation. At the physiological level, we wish to know what stimuli lead to the secretion of the hormone from the endocrine gland, what the physiological effects of the hormone are on target tissues, and how the response to hormone enables the organism as a whole to adapt to the original stimulus. At a more biochemical level, an important question is that of how the hormone acts on target cells—what are the receptors, do enzyme activities or amounts alter in response to hormone, and what other changes occur at the chemical level? It is also valuable to know how the hormone is eventually removed from the circulation and destroyed.

Most of what is known about the action of hormones has come from the study of mammals, in particular, man and laboratory rodents. Much of this chapter is devoted to a consideration of mammalian hormones, but it should be realized that, even within the mammals, species-specific differences occur in the importance of different hormones.

Mammalian hormones

Mammalian hormones belong to one of three chemical types—peptides, steroids or amino-acid derivatives. The peptide hormones, and some of the amino-acid derivatives such as adrenaline, affect target cells through receptors at the plasma membrane, whereas lipid-soluble steroid hormones enter the cell and act through intracellular receptors.

The hormones which act through plasma membrane receptors bring about most, if not all, of their effects by means of intracellular regulatory substances known as *second messengers*; for example, a number of hormones are known to act by altering (usually elevating) the concentration of cyclic AMP in target cells. Although cyclic AMP is the best-

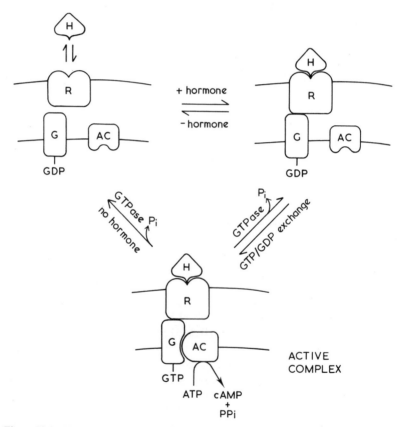

Figure 10.1 Hormonal activation of adenylate cyclase. Hormone (H) binds to a receptor (R) on the outer surface of the plasma membrane, and a signal is transmitted to the nucleotide binding protein (G), either by a conformational change (as represented here) or by some other mechanism. GTP then exchanges for GDP, and the GTP form of the nucleotide-binding protein activates adenylate cyclase (AC). GTPase continuously reverses the activation.

established second messenger of hormone action, some hormones probably operate through other regulatory signals, of which calcium ions and perhaps cyclic GMP are the best candidates.

The sequence of events by which hormones act on cyclic AMP is shown in figure 10.1. In a non-stimulated ("resting") cell, it is likely that the two membrane components of the system, receptor and adenylate cyclase, are not specifically associated together. When the hormone binds to its receptor, a change in receptor conformation, or a perturbation of the membrane ensues such that the adenylate cyclase activity is affected.

The adenylate cyclase consists of two types of subunit, one of which is catalytic (C in the figure) and the second of which is a nucleotide-binding subunit (G in the figure). When the nucleotide-binding subunit binds GTP, then the catalytic subunit becomes active and is able to synthesize cyclic AMP. The binding of GTP is believed to be promoted when a stimulating hormone binds to its receptor. However, another component of the adenylate cyclase system catalyses hydrolysis of GTP to GDP, and the resulting GDP-enzyme is inactive in synthesis of cyclic AMP (figure 10.1). In other words, there is a cycle of reactions by which the adenylate cyclase always tends to revert to an inactive form, and only remains significantly active in the continued presence of activating hormone-receptor complex.

As a result of adenylate cyclase activation, the cyclic AMP concentration in the cytosol of the stimulated cell is increased. The main effect of this elevated cyclic AMP is believed to be on the activation of cyclic AMP-dependent protein kinase. In the resting cell, the protein kinase is present as an inactive complex of catalytic and regulatory subunits.

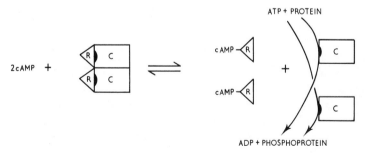

Figure 10.2 Activation of cyclic AMP-dependent protein kinase. Cyclic AMP binds to the regulatory subunits (R) and causes dissociation of the protein kinase complex to give active catalytic subunits (C) which can then catalyse phosphorylation of target proteins such as phosphorylase *b* kinase.

Binding of cyclic AMP to the regulatory subunits promotes dissociation of the complex, to leave the catalytic subunits in their active forms (figure 10.2). The cyclic AMP-dependent protein kinase then catalyses the phosphorylation of regulatory enzymes and other regulatory proteins within the cell to effect the changes in activity which are the ultimate targets of hormone action. For example, hormonal control of glycogen metabolism is achieved through phosphorylation of phosphorylase b kinase and of glycogen synthase (p. 122).

All of these activating reactions are opposed by other reactions which tend to return the system to the resting state, when hormonal stimulation ceases. Adenylate cyclase becomes inactive by virtue of its GTPase activity, cyclic AMP is hydrolysed to AMP by a phosphodiesterase, dissociation of the cyclic AMP-regulator protein occurs at low cyclic AMP concentrations, and the regulatory proteins are dephosphorylated by specific phosphatases.

A number of different hormones activate the cyclic AMP system, and yet each has a different and characteristic effect in the animal. This specificity of different hormones acting through the same second-messenger system is achieved in two ways. Firstly, the hormone can only activate cells which have the appropriate receptor for that hormone, so cells are programmed to respond to only certain hormones according to their characteristic complement of receptors. Secondly, different cells have different substrates, or combinations of substrates, available for phosphorylation by protein kinase; for example, in fat cells the main substrate for cyclic AMP-dependent protein kinase is a hormone-sensitive lipase, whereas in muscle it is phosphorylase b kinase and glycogen synthetase. Consequently, hormonal elevation of cyclic AMP in fat cells increases fat breakdown, but in liver increases glycogen breakdown.

Steroid hormones do not appear to operate through a second-messenger system. They enter cells and bind to intracellular protein receptors in the cytoplasm. The receptor-hormone complex is then taken up by the nucleus, where it promotes the synthesis of selected messenger RNA molecules. The cell then proceeds to synthesize the particular group of proteins coded for by the new messenger RNAs, and which are characteristic of the action of the hormone. Again, the ability of a tissue to respond to a hormone depends on the presence of the appropriate receptor in the cell.

For most hormones, amplification of the initial hormone signal is achieved by the presence of catalytic stages between hormone binding and the final effect. This permits a single hormone molecule to affect the metabolism of many substrate molecules, for example, a molecule of hormone by activating a single adenylate cyclase molecule can bring about the synthesis of many molecules of cyclic AMP. For each protein kinase molecule thus activated, many protein molecules can be phosphorylated. Similarly for steroid hormones—each hormone molecule may activate the synthesis of a number of messenger RNA molecules, each of which can code for the synthesis of many protein molecules.

Glucagon

The islets of Langerhans in the pancreas are endocrine glands which secrete two major peptide hormones of fundamental importance to the regulation of carbohydrate metabolism. These hormones are insulin and glucagon, and each is secreted by different groups of cells: the A cells (or "α cells") secrete glucagon, and the B cells ("β cells") secrete insulin.

The main effect of glucagon is to promote glucose release from the liver into the blood by the stimulation of glycogen breakdown to glucose, and by the stimulation of gluconeogenesis. Glucagon action is therefore of particular importance during periods when insufficient food is available and the animal has to rely on its reserves to maintain blood glucose at normal concentrations (p. 182).

The rate of release of glucagon from the A cells is regulated by a number of factors (table 10.1). Of particular importance is the effect of low plasma glucose concentrations, which increase glucagon release and thus stimulate glucose production and help to restore normal plasma glucose concentrations.

Most of the effects of glucagon on its target tissues are mediated by

Table 10.1 Factors which affect the rates of secretion of pancreatic hormones.

	Stimulators	*Inhibitors*
A. *Glucagon*	noradrenaline amino acids growth hormone	glucose insulin somatostatin
B. *Insulin*	glucose, mannose amino acids (e.g. leucine) gut peptides (e.g. G.I.P.) glucagon adrenaline (β-receptors) agents which elevate cyclic AMP (e.g. caffeine) acetylcholine	somatostatin

elevation of cyclic AMP within the cell. In the liver, this results in a phosphorylation of phosphorylase b kinase, with consequent conversion of phosphorylase b to a as described on p. 122. Glycogen synthase will be converted to its less active phosphorylated form, so that the overall effect of glucagon is to stimulate glycogen breakdown and inhibit its synthesis.

The mechanism by which glucagon stimulates gluconeogenesis is not so clearly established. It is probable that inhibition of glycolysis may be as important as specific stimulation of gluconeogenic enzymes. Thus the flow of substrate through the competing pathways of glycolysis and gluconeogenesis depends on the relative rates of the reactions which bring about recycling of substrates through opposing reactions of the two pathways (p. 65). Figure 10.3 shows how recycling of pyruvate and of fructose phosphates occurs.

During pyruvate recycling, if the rate of the pyruvate kinase reaction is decreased without affecting the rate of the other reactions of the cycle, then the net result is an increased flow of substrate in the gluconeogenic direction. In accordance with this, it has recently been found that the L-type pyruvate kinase of liver can be phosphorylated by cyclic AMP-dependent protein kinase, and that such phosphorylation leads to a

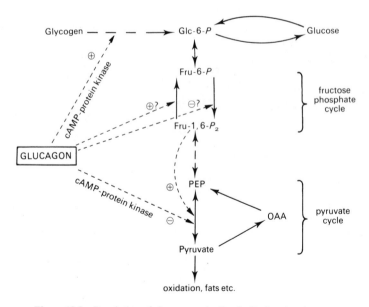

Figure 10.3   Regulation of glucose production in the liver by glucagon.

decrease in enzymic activity. This effect can therefore partly account for the observed stimulation of gluconeogenesis by glucagon.

Glucagon also seems to affect the cycling of substrate between fructose phosphates such that fructose 6-phosphate formation is favoured. Fructose bisphosphatase is converted by phosphorylation to a more active form, although the physiological importance of this effect is not as well established as for pyruvate kinase. There is also evidence that phosphofructokinase is inhibited by some unknown mechanism in glucagon-treated cells. A change in activity of either of these enzymes could explain the observed decrease in concentration of fructose 1,6-bisphosphate which results from exposure of liver cells to glucagon. This decrease in fructose bisphosphate will reinforce the inhibition of pyruvate kinase, since the L-type pyruvate kinase is only fully active in the presence of high concentrations of fructose bisphosphate.

Glucagon may also affect adipose tissue by stimulating triglyceride breakdown and subsequent release of fatty acids into the blood. Although this response of adipose tissue to glucagon is different from that of liver, the physiological function is similar: the availability of fat substrates allows many tissues to metabolize lipids as an energy source in place of glucose. This has a sparing effect on the rate of removal of glucose from the circulation, and hence decreases the rate at which the liver needs to supply glucose to the blood. This effect of glucagon on adipose tissue may be physiologically less important than effects on the liver, at least in some animal species. Thus glucagon is secreted into the portal vein and reaches the liver in fairly high concentration, but since the liver is also a major site of inactivation of glucagon, the concentration of the hormone reaching the rest of the circulation is relatively low.

The effects of glucagon described above all occur rapidly, within a minute or two of exposure of a tissue to the hormone. In addition, glucagon has slower effects on tissues which are brought about by changing the rate of synthesis of certain enzymes and thus altering the total amount of such enzymes in the cell. The gluconeogenic enzyme phosphoenolpyruvate carboxykinase is increased in amount when liver is exposed to glucagon.

Insulin

The insulin molecule consists of two peptide chains linked by disulphide bridges. It is synthesized in the B cells of the islets of Langerhans and stored in vesicles as a complex with zinc ions.

Insulin secretion from B cells is regulated by a number of different factors (table 10.1), of which the most important physiologically is probably the plasma glucose concentration. The molecular mechanism by which insulin secretion is controlled is not known in detail. Calcium ions are required, and elevated cyclic AMP concentrations in the B cells stimulate secretion. It is likely that microtubules are involved in moving secretory vesicles to the cell surface, and that these are activated during the secretory process.

Insulin has a number of effects on target tissues, all of which can be considered to be anabolic. Thus it stimulates the uptake of glucose by muscle, adipose tissue and a number of other tissues, and it promotes conversion of glucose into storage products (glycogen in muscle and liver, triglycerides in adipose tissue). Insulin also stimulates amino-acid uptake and protein synthesis, and inhibits the breakdown of glycogen, triglycerides and proteins. All of these anabolic effects of insulin are related to the physiological requirements of the animal after intake of a meal, when the products of digestion must be metabolized and converted to storage products and cell materials.

Some of the effects of insulin on tissues take place much more rapidly than others. Rapid effects occur within a few minutes of exposure of a tissue to insulin, and include the stimulation of glucose transport and activation of glycogen and lipid synthesis. Slower effects of insulin are on rates of protein synthesis, and these may take an hour or more to take effect. Insulin also promotes alterations in the amounts of certain enzymes in tissues, such as an increase in glucokinase in the liver. These effects are also rather slow.

For its action on target cells, insulin must first bind to specific glycoproteins of the outer surface of the plasma membrane. How the occupation of these receptors brings about effects on cells is still not understood. Various second messengers have been proposed to transmit the signal produced by hormone-receptor interaction to the cell interior, but none can account for all of the different effects of insulin on tissues. In some systems, insulin prevents the elevation of cyclic AMP caused by glucagon or adrenaline, but this effect is not always found, and insulin alone does not depress resting levels of cyclic AMP. Insulin generally opposes the effects of hormones which elevate cyclic AMP, and may do this by producing an inhibitor which prevents activation of cyclic AMP-dependent protein kinase. Other candidates considered for a second messenger have been cyclic GMP or calcium ions. However, although insulin can elevate the concentrations of one or other of these in some systems, these are by no means universal effects, and are likely to be secondary to a more direct effect of insulin on another (unknown) factor.

Intracellular proteins have been found which bind insulin with high affinity, and it has been suggested that the slower effects of insulin could be the result of insulin entry into cells and its interaction with such intracellular receptors. These proposals are not generally accepted, however, and at the present time it seems most likely that all of the effects of insulin are initiated as a result of its binding to the cell surface receptors.

In keeping with its role as a rapid-acting hormone, insulin is not only released quickly but is also destroyed quickly, and has a half-life in the circulation of less than thirty minutes. It is removed by the liver, kidneys and muscles. Two mechanisms exist for its inactivation. In the first, a glutathione-dependent protein-disulphide reductase catalyses reduction of the disulphide bridges of insulin, and so separates it into its component A and B chains, which are themselves hormonally inactive. In the second mechanism, the insulin is destroyed proteolytically, perhaps after first binding to its specific cell-surface receptors.

Adrenaline and noradrenaline

Adrenaline (epinephrine) and noradrenaline (norepinephrine) are catecholamines derived from tyrosine (figure 10.4). The endocrine source of adrenaline is the adrenal medulla, from which it is secreted rapidly into the blood in response to stress or an immediate physical threat to the animal. Its physiological effects (elevation of heart rate and blood pressure, increase of blood glucose, etc.) help to prepare the animal for physical action. Noradrenaline is also secreted by the adrenal medulla, but is perhaps more important as a transmitter of the sympathetic nervous system. It is released locally at target tissues so that concentrations are only elevated significantly at the site of action. Despite these differences in release and delivery to target tissues, it is convenient to consider the catecholamines together, because they act on the same receptor systems in cells.

There are two classes of catecholamine receptor which differ from each other in the way in which the hormonal effect is transmitted. The β-receptors act through the adenylate cyclase system, so cells with this type of receptor respond to catecholamines by elevation of cyclic AMP, activation of protein kinase, and phosphorylation of regulatory proteins. However, the α-receptors have no direct effect on the cyclic AMP system. Stimulation of α-receptors causes elevation of calcium ion concentrations

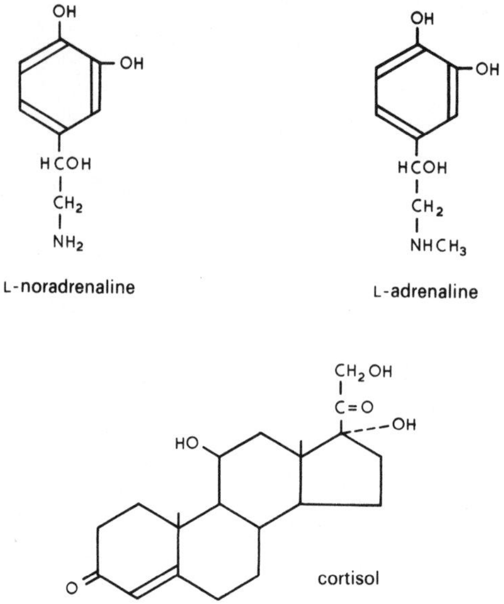

Figure 10.4   Structures of some vertebrate hormones.

in the cytosol, either by increasing the permeability of the plasma membrane to calcium and allowing entry of extracellular calcium, or by releasing calcium from an intracellular site, perhaps the plasma membrane or mitochondria, where calcium is sequestered as "trigger calcium". Some cells, such as those of liver, have both α- and β-receptors, which makes interpretation of the effects of catecholamines on them rather difficult.

The catecholamines have several effects on carbohydrate metabolism. Like glucagon, they stimulate glucose release from the liver by stimulating glycogenolysis and gluconeogenesis. Stimulation of β-receptors elevates cyclic AMP and promotes glycogenolysis via phosphorylation of phosphorylase b kinase. However, this is probably less important in most mammalian species than the effect on α-receptors, which by elevation of calcium ion concentrations stimulate phosphorylase b kinase (p. 124). Physiologically it is likely that local release of noradrenaline from the sympathetic nerves is the most important catecholamine effect on liver, since levels of circulating catecholamines rarely achieve a concentration sufficiently high to have a marked effect on liver. Another effect of catecholamines is on muscle, where both glycogenolysis and the transport of glucose into muscle is stimulated. This supplies the muscle with more substrate for contraction.

The glucocorticoids

Steroid hormones originating from the adrenal cortex fall into two main categories—those that exert an effect mainly on ion balance, and those with effects on the metabolism of glucose and other substrates. This division between the two groups is not complete, as hormones with a strong effect on ion balance usually have a weaker effect on substrate metabolism and *vice versa*. The metabolic steroids of the adrenal cortex are known as the glucocorticoids, and cortisol (figure 10.4) is the most potent of these.

The glucocorticoids are relatively slowly-acting hormones, whose main effect seems to be on the rates of synthesis of certain enzymes. The effect of glucocorticoids on liver is to increase the amounts of enzymes concerned with gluconeogenesis (in particular, phosphoenolpyruvate carboxykinase) and amino-acid degradation (tyrosine aminotransferase, glutamylalanine aminotransferase, serine dehydratase). Glucose 6-phosphatase activity is elevated by glucocorticoids. The effect on muscle and a number of other tissues is to promote protein breakdown and to inhibit glucose uptake. The overall physiological effects of glucocorticoids are therefore to increase blood glucose concentrations by gluconeogenesis from substrates provided by breakdown of extrahepatic proteins.

Glucocorticoid action is particularly associated with conditions of stress. Thus the concentrations of glucocorticoids in the blood are elevated by injury, disease, exposure to cold, hard exercise, starvation, and mental stress caused by anxiety.

Other hormones

Several other hormones are known to affect carbohydrate metabolism, and these may become important under some physiological conditions; for example, growth hormone elevates the concentration of glucose in the blood, and this effect is mediated partly by stimulation of glucagon release. Thyroid hormones can also indirectly affect carbohydrate metabolism by increasing the number of catecholamine receptors in cells and thus increasing the response of cells to catecholamines.

Another indirect regulator of carbohydrate metabolism may be somatostatin. This is a peptide, originally found in the hypophysis, which controls the release of growth hormone (somatotropin) from the anterior pituitary. More recently somatostatin has also been found in the islets of Langerhans where it is synthesized in the D cells. Somatostatin inhibits the release of both insulin and glucagon, and has been used experimentally and even clinically for this purpose. Local release of somatostatin could therefore regulate the secretion of the pancreatic hormones, but it is not yet clear how this mechanism operates physiologically.

The pituitary hormones vasopressin and angiotensin can stimulate the release of glucose from the liver. Their action resembles that of catecholamines acting through α-receptors—they elevate intracellular calcium and stimulate glycogenolysis. These effects are unlikely to be of physiological importance under most conditions, but may become so under conditions of great stress. Thus when a haemorrhage (large loss of blood) takes place, the blood pressure drops and large quantities of vasopressin and angiotensin are released. The resulting increase in blood glucose may be valuable to survival under these conditions.

Physiological regulation of blood glucose concentrations

The concentration of glucose in the blood of most mammals is regulated within very narrow limits of between 4 and 6 mM. This control is maintained despite wide variations in the rate at which glucose enters and leaves the blood. During digestion of a large meal, the rate of glucose absorption increases enormously, yet the blood concentration rises by only a relatively modest amount because of increased uptake by tissues. Similarly, during vigorous exercise, the extraction of glucose by muscles increases rapidly, but there is little change in the concentration of blood glucose, because the increased uptake is balanced by output from the liver. In contrast to this well-regulated system, the concentrations of other metabolites in blood may alter by much larger amounts. Lactate concentrations vary by tenfold or more, and ketone bodies by more than one hundred times.

This careful regulation of glucose concentration is important to maintain normal function. Concentrations below 3 mM are too low to supply the brain with sufficient glucose, and hypoglycaemic coma occurs at such concentrations. On the other hand, concentrations of glucose above 8 to 10 mM exceed the capacity of the kidneys to reabsorb the sugar from the glomerular filtrate, so glucose is lost to the urine (a condition known as glycosuria).

The two main hormones responsible for regulating blood glucose

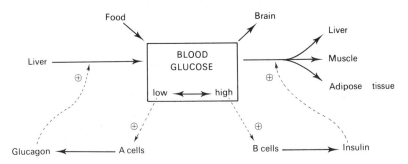

Figure 10.5   The role of pancreatic hormones in balancing glucose flow into and out of the blood. For simplicity, inhibitory effects and other hormones have been omitted.

concentrations are glucagon and insulin, and the release of both is subject to a complex series of controls (table 10.1). Figure 10.5 shows the main features of the relationship between blood glucose and the release of glucagon and insulin.

During assimilation of a meal, the products of digestion increase in concentration, and the glucose and amino acids stimulate insulin secretion from the B cells of the pancreas. In addition, regulatory peptides are secreted by the gut very soon after food intake, and these have a rapid effect in stimulating insulin release, even before blood glucose levels are affected. The elevated glucose and insulin then suppress glucagon secretion, so that the insulin/glucagon ratio is high. The tissues (muscle, liver, adipose tissue) respond by converting glucose to glycogen and lipids, and at the same time glucose and fatty-acid release is inhibited. Later, as food digestion approaches completion, the ratio of insulin/glucagon decreases until eventually the balance of metabolism is changed towards net glucose release from the liver to maintain the blood sugar level.

During short periods of starvation (24 to 48 hours), there is a heavy reliance on glucose supply from the liver. Plasma insulin levels decrease, and this limits glucose uptake by peripheral tissues. However, the brain is not sensitive to insulin and still uses large quantities of glucose—about 70% of the total blood glucose in man, but less in animals with proportionally smaller brains. Lower insulin levels also relieve insulin inhibition of glycogenolysis and gluconeogenesis in liver, and of lipolysis in adipose tissue. Glucagon concentrations increase as a result of lower blood glucose levels and low insulin concentrations (insulin inhibits glucagon release). The glucagon promotes glucose secretion from the liver and, to a lesser extent, fatty-acid production by adipose tissue. Gluco-corticoids are released, and these increase protein breakdown in a number of tissues and thus supply the liver with increased gluconeogenic substrates. There is also an increase in amount of some gluconeogenic enzymes as a result of the decrease in insulin and increase in gluco-corticoids and glucagon. As starvation progresses, the liver starts to convert an increasing amount of fatty acids into ketone bodies (β-hydroxybutyrate and acetoacetate) which can be used as fuels by other tissues, especially the heart.

During long-term starvation, gluconeogenesis actually decreases again as many tissues, including the brain, gradually adapt to using ketone bodies as fuels in place of glucose. The concentration of ketone bodies in blood during long-term starvation may be about 6 mM—about 100 times that in the well-fed state.

During muscular exercise, the increased utilization of glucose by the muscles is compensated for by an increase in glucose production by the liver. This is brought about partly by an increase in sympathetic stimulation of the liver which increases glycogenolysis, mainly through an effect on the α-receptors. Glucagon concentrations also increase, probably as a result of sympathetic stimulation of the A cells and any decrease that may occur in the concentration of glucose in the plasma. During longer periods of exercise, other hormones become involved—insulin decreases, and glucocorticoids and growth hormone concentrations increase.

Diabetes

Diabetes mellitus is a disease in which the concentration of glucose in blood is abnormally high. One cause of diabetes is a lack of insulin as a result of damage to the B-cells of the pancreas. Often the numbers of insulin-secreting cells are abnormally low, and the numbers of glucagon-secreting A-cells are high. Other causes of diabetes common in older individuals include defects in the ability of B-cells to respond to increased glucose concentrations, or decreased sensitivity of target cells to normal insulin levels.

There are gradations in the severity of the disease, varying from an almost complete lack of circulating insulin, common in individuals who first show symptoms when young, to a partial lack of insulin which is more typically found in maturity-onset cases. It has been estimated that up to 5 % of all humans are affected by the disease sooner or later in their life. Although diabetes is not directly inherited, some individuals are genetically at greater risk of developing the disease than others. The chances of developing diabetes are also higher in obese persons.

In diabetics, the blood glucose concentrations are usually higher than normal at all times, but become excessively high during the digestion of a carbohydrate meal, so that the renal threshold for glucose is exceeded and glucose appears in the urine. In severe cases, the renal threshold for glucose is exceeded at all times, and sugar is excreted continuously.

In the absence of insulin, many cells are unable to take up or metabolize glucose at a normal rate, so that glucose utilization is impaired and there is a heavier reliance on lipid substrates for metabolic fuels, despite an ample supply of carbohydrate from food. The concentrations of fatty acids, and particularly ketone bodies, in the blood increase as a result of the low insulin concentration which permits increased rates of lipolysis and ketone body formation to take place. Often quantities of ketone bodies are excreted in the urine, and the pH of the blood falls as a result of the high concentration of acetoacetate and β-hydroxybutyrate. Gluconeogenesis is stimulated, and tissues become wasted as protein degradation (normally inhibited by insulin) occurs and supplies gluconeogenic substrate.

These effects are not only due to a lack of insulin, but are made worse by the increased levels of glucagon which are usually found in diabetics. This may be caused by a lack of the normal inhibitory influence of insulin on glucagon release.

A more rare condition is that of hypoglycaemia, in which the blood glucose concentrations are abnormally low. One cause of hypoglycaemia is the development of insulin tumours where excessive insulin production occurs. Hypoglycaemia can also occur temporarily in diabetics when an inappropriately high dose of insulin is administered to the patient.

Invertebrate hormones

Regulation of metabolism, development and growth is as important in invertebrates as it is in vertebrates. The most widely studied group of invertebrates is the insects, where the general chemical types of hormones are similar to those of mammals.

Rapid effects on the metabolism of insects have been shown for a group of peptide hormones secreted from the corpora cardiaca (neurohaemal glands in the head), for example, blow-flies secrete a hyperglycaemic peptide hormone into the blood during flight. This acts on the fat body (which in insects combines the functions of liver and adipose tissue) and stimulates the conversion of stored glycogen reserves to the blood sugar, trehalose. The trehalose then provides substrate for the flight muscles. The hyperglycaemic hormone of insects therefore resembles glucagon of mammals in some of its effects. Like glucagon, it appears to act through elevation of intracellular cyclic AMP and activation of phosphorylase. There is also evidence that some insects possess a hypoglycaemic hormone which decreases trehalose levels in the blood, and in this respect is comparable with the insulin of mammals.

Plant hormones

In animals, hormones are secreted by specialized endocrine glands, but in plants there are no such glands. Instead, plant hormones or growth substances are secreted by non-specialized tissues. The main effects of such substances at the physiological level are upon plant growth, but little is known of their molecular mechanism of action.

The best-established effect of plant growth substances on carbohydrate metabolism is in the germination of cereal seeds. In such seeds, germination is initiated after the uptake of water. The embryo then becomes active and secretes one of a group of plant hormones known as the *gibberellins*. In barley, the gibberellin GA_3 is most important. The main targets for gibberellin action are the cells of the aleurone layer. These cells surround the endosperm, which contains the main store of starch reserves destined to supply the embryo with nutrient during growth into a seedling. The effect of gibberellins on the aleurone cells is to stimulate them to synthesize and release enzymes required to hydrolyse the stored nutrients. Enzymes which are synthesized after treatment of aleurone cells with gibberellins include α-amylase, α-glucosidase, limit dextrinases, β-glucanase and proteinase, all of which are secreted into the endosperm. There is a delay of 8 hours or more before enzyme secretion starts, and this may represent the time required for synthesis of messenger RNAs to manufacture the proteins.

Gibberellins indirectly affect the activity of β-amylase in the sub-aleurone layer. This enzyme is entirely synthesized during grain development, but is present largely in an inactive form complexed with protein. Gibberellins bring about the activation of β-amylase by inducing enzymes which reduce disulphide bridges between β-amylase and complexed protein, and by inducing proteinases which may attack the complexed protein.

FURTHER READING

General

The following series are useful sources of reviews:

Advances in Carbohydrate Chemistry and Biochemistry
Annual Review of Biochemistry
Annual Review of Microbiology
Annual Review of Physiology
Annual Review of Plant Physiology
Current Topics in Cellular Regulation
Essays in Biochemistry
MTP International Review of Biochemistry
Trends in Biochemical Sciences ("TIBS")

Chapter 1

Bentley, R. (1972) "Configurational and Conformational Aspects of Carbohydrate Biochemistry", *Ann. Rev. Biochem.*, **41**, 953–996.

Coffey, S. (ed.) (1967) *Rodd's Chemistry of Carbon Compounds* Vol. **1F**, Elsevier, Amsterdam.

Ferrier, R. J. and Collins, P. M. (1972) *Monosaccharide Chemistry*, Penguin Books, Middlesex.

IUPAC-IUB Commission (1971) "Tentative Rules for Carbohydrate Nomenclature", see e.g. *Biochem. J.*, **125**, 673–695.

Pigman, W. and Horton, D. (1971) *The Carbohydrates: Chemistry and Biochemistry*, 2nd edition, (3 vols.) Academic Press, New York.

Stoddart, J. F. (1971) *Stereochemistry of Carbohydrates*, John Wiley & Sons, New York.

Chapter 2

Atkinson, D. E. (1977) *Cellular Energy Metabolism*, Academic Press, New York.

Benkovic, S. J. and Schray, K. J. (1976) "The Anomeric Specificity of Glycolytic Enzymes", *Advan. Enzymol.*, **44**, 139–164.

Boyer, P. D. (ed.) *The Enzymes*, 3rd edition, Academic Press, New York. (A series with articles on individual enzymes).

Clark, M. G. and Lardy, H. A. (1975) "Regulation of Intermediary Carbohydrate Metabolism", *MTP International Rev. Biochem*, **5**, 223–266.

Gottschalk, G. and Andreeson, J. R. (1979) "Energy Metabolism in Anaerobes", *MTP International Rev. Biochem.*, **21**, 25–57.

Krebs, H. A. (1972) "The Pasteur Effect and the Relations between Respiration and Fermentation", *Essays in Biochem.*, **8**, 1–34.

Newsholme, E. A. and Start, C. (1973) *Regulation in Metabolism*, John Wiley & Sons, London.

Uyeda, K. (1979) "Phosphofructokinase", *Advan. Enzymol.*, **48**, 193–224.

187

Chapter 3

Barnett, J. E. G. and Corina, D. L. (1972) "Sugars Specifically Labelled with Isotopes of Hydrogen", *Advan. Carbohydrate Chem. Biochem.*, **27**, 127–190. (Interconversion of sugars).

Cooper, R. A. (1978) "Intermediary Metabolism of Monosaccharides by Bacteria", *MTP International Rev. Biochem.*, **16**, 37–73.

Eggleston, L. V. and Krebs, H. A. (1974) "Regulation of the Pentose Phosphate Cycle", *Biochem. J.*, **138**, 425–435.

Gabriel, O. and Van Lenton, L. (1978) "The Interconversion of Monosaccharides", *MTP International Rev. Biochem.*, **16**, 1–36.

Gander, J. E. (1976) "Mono- and Oligosaccharides", in *Plant Biochemistry*, 3rd edition (ed. Bonner, J. and Varner, J. E.), Academic Press, New York, 337–380.

Hanson, R. W. and Mehlman, M. A. (eds.) (1976) *Gluconeogenesis: its Regulation in Mammalian Species*, John Wiley & Sons, New York. (Reviews).

King, C. G. and Burns, J. J. (eds.) (1975) "2nd Conference on Vitamin C", *Annals New York Acad. Sci.*, **258**. (Reviews).

Michell, R. H. (1979) "Inositol Phospholipids in Membrane Function", *Trends in Biochem. Sci.*, **4**, 128–131.

Pauling, L. C. (1976) *Vitamin C, the Common Cold and the Flu*, Freeman & Co., San Francisco.

Chapter 4

Barber, J. (ed.) (1976) *The Intact Chloroplast*, Elsevier, Amsterdam. (Reviews).

Bassham, J. A. and Calvin, M. (1957) *The Path of Carbon in Photosynthesis*, Englewood Cliffs University Press.

Bonner, J. D. and Varner, J. E. (eds.) (1976) *Plant Biochemistry*, 3rd edition, Academic Press, New York (e.g. articles by Kok and Hatch).

Doelle, H. W. (1975) *Bacterial Metabolism*, 2nd edition, Academic Press, New York, chapter 3.

Gibbs, M. and Latzko, E. (eds.) (1979) "Photosynthesis 2", *Encyclopedia of Plant Physiology: New Series* Vol. **6**, Springer-Verlag, Berlin. (Reviews).

Hatch, M. D. (1978) "Regulation of Enzymes in C_4 Photosynthesis", *Current Topics in Cell. Regulation*, **14**, 1–27.

Whittingham, C. P. (1974) *The Mechanism of Photosynthesis*, Edward Arnold, London.

Chapter 5

Crane, R. K. (1976) "The Gradient Hypothesis and Other Models of Carrier-Mediated Active Transport", *Rev. Physiol. Biochem. Pharmacol.*, **78**, 99–159.

Dahlqvist, A. (1978) "Disturbances of the Digestion and Absorption of Carbohydrates", *MTP International Rev. Biochem.*, **16**, 179–207.

Rosen, B. P. (ed.) (1978) *Bacterial Transport*, Marcel Dekker, New York, Basel. (Reviews).

Tristram, M. (1978) "Transport of Organic Solutes by Bacteria", in *Companion to Microbiology*, **4**, (ed. Bull, A. T. and Meadow, P. H.) Longman, London, 297–320.

Wilson, D. B. (1978) "Cellular Transport Mechanisms", *Ann. Rev. Biochem.*, **47**, 933–965.

Chapter 6

Chen, M. and Whistler, R. L. (1977) "Metabolism of D-Fructose", *Advan. Carbohydrate Chem. Biochem.*, **34**, 285–343.

Elbein, A. D. (1974) "The Metabolism of α,α-Trehalose", *Advan. Carbohydrate Chem. Biochem.*, **30**, 227–256.

Pontis, H. G. (1977) "Riddle of Sucrose", *MTP International Rev. Biochem.*, **13**, 79–117.

Yudkin, J., Edelman, J. and Hough, L. (eds.) (1971) *Sugar*, Butterworths, London. (Sucrose chemistry, biochemistry, relation to disease).

Chapter 7

ap Rees, T. (1974) "Pathways of Carbohydrate Breakdown in Higher Plants", *MTP International Rev. Biochem.*, **11**, 89–127.

Banks, W. and Greenwood, C. T. (1975) *Starch and its Components*, Edinburgh University Press.

Blanshard, J. M. V. and Mitchell, J. R. (eds.) (1979) *Polysaccharides in Food*, Butterworths, London. (Reviews).

Busby, S. J. W. and Radda, G. K. (1976) "The Glycogen Phosphorylase System", *Current Topics in Cell. Regulation*, **10**, 89–160.

Cohen, P. (1976) *Control of Enzyme Activity*, Chapman & Hall, London.

French, D. (1975) "Chemistry and Biochemistry of Starch", *MTP International Rev. Biochem.*, **5**, 267–335.

Griffiths, J. R. and Rahim, Z. H. A. (1978) "Glycogen as a Fuel for Skeletal Muscle", *Biochem. Soc. Trans.*, **6**, 530–534.

Howell, R. R. (1978) "The Glycogen Storage Diseases" in *The Metabolic Basis of Inherited Disease*, (ed. Stanbury, J. B., Wyngaarden, J. B. and Fredrickson, D. S.) McGraw-Hill, New York, 137–159.

Krebs, E. G. and Priess, J. (1975) "Regulatory Mechanisms in Glycogen Metabolism", *MTP International Rev. Biochem.*, **5**, 337–389.

Rees, D. A. (1977) *Polysaccharide Shapes*, Chapman & Hall, London.

Stitt, M. Bulpin, P. V. and ap Rees, T. (1978) "Pathway of Starch Breakdown in Photosynthetic Tissues of *Pisum sativum*", *Biochim. Biophys. Acta*, **544**, 200–214.

Turner, J. F. and Turner, D. H. (1975) "The Regulation of Carbohydrate Metabolism", *Ann. Rev. Plant Physiol.*, **26**, 159–186.

Chapter 8

Albersheim, P. (1975) "The Walls of Growing Plant Cells", *Scientific American*, **232**, (4), 80–95.

Albersheim, P. (1978) "Structure and Biosynthesis of the Primary Cell Walls of Plants", *MTP International Rev. Biochem.*, **16**, 127–150.

Comper, W. D. and Laurent, T. C. (1978) "Physiological Function of Connective Tissue Polysaccharides", *Physiol. Rev.* **58**, 255–315.

Ghuysen, J-M. (1977) "Biosynthesis and Assembly of Bacterial Cell Walls", in *The Synthesis, Assembly and Turnover of Cell Surface Components*, (ed. Poste, G. and Nicolson, G. L.) North Holland, Amsterdam, 463–595.

Horowitz, M. and Pigman, W. (eds.) (1977–8) *The Glycoconjugates* (2 vols.) Academic Press, New York. (Reviews relevant to Chapters 8 and 9).

Hopp, H. E., Romero, P. A., Daleo, G. P. and Pont Lezica, R. (1978) "Synthesis of Cellulose Precursors. The Involvement of Lipid-linked Sugars", *Eur. J. Biochem.*, **84**, 561–571.

Lindahl, U. and Höök, M. (1978) "Glycosaminoglycans and their Binding to Biological Macromolecules", *Ann. Rev. Biochem.*, **47**, 385–417.

McKusick, V. A., Neufeld, E. F. and Kelly, T. F. (1978) "The Mucopolysaccharide Storage Diseases", in *The Metabolic Basis of Inherited Disease*, (ed. Stanbury, J. B., Wyngaarden, J. B. and Fredrickson, D. S.) McGraw-Hill, New York, 1282–1307.

Muir, H. and Hardingham, T. E. (1975) "Structure of Proteoglycans", *MTP International Rev. Biochem.*, **5**, 153–222.

Preston, R. D. (1974) *The Physical Biology of Plant Cell Walls*, Chapman & Hall, London.

Preston, R. D. (1979) "Polysaccharide Conformation and Cell Wall Function", *Ann. Rev. Plant Physiol.*, **30**, 55–78.

Strominger, J. L. (1975) "The Actions of Penicillins and Other Antibiotics on Bacterial Cell Wall Synthesis", *MTP International Rev. Biochem.*, **2**, 207–227.

Tomasz, A. (1979) "The Mechanism of the Irreversible Antimicrobial Effects of Penicillins", *Ann. Rev. Microbiol.*, **33**, 113–137.

Chapter 9

Ashwell, G. and Morell, A. G. (1974) "The Role of Surface Carbohydrates in Hepatocyte Recognition of Circulating Glycoproteins", *Advan. Enzymol.*, **41**, 99–128.

Brady, R. O. (1978) "Sphingolipidoses", *Ann. Rev. Biochem.*, **47**, 687–713.

Curtis, A. (ed.) (1978) *Cell–Cell Recognition*, Symp. Soc. Exp. Biol., **32**. (Reviews).

Feeney, R. E. (1978) "Antifreeze Proteins from Fish Bloods", *Advan. Protein Chem.*, **32**, 191–282.

Flowers, H. M. and Sharon, N. (1979) "Glycosidases—Properties and Application to Study of Complex Carbohydrates and Cell Surfaces", *Advan. Enzymol.*, **48**, 29–95.

Goldstein, I. J. and Hayes, C. E. (1978) "The Lectins: Carbohydrate-Binding Proteins of Plants and Animals", *Advan. Carbohydrate Chem. Biochem.*, **35**, 127–340.

Hughes, R. C. (1976) *Membrane Glycoproteins*, Butterworths, London.

Jamieson, G. A. and Robinson, D. M. (eds.) (1977) *Mammalian Cell Membranes*, Vol. 4, Butterworths, London. (Reviews).

Jeljaszewicz, J. and Wadstrom, T. (eds.) (1978) *Bacterial Toxins and Cell Membranes*, Academic Press, London. (Reviews).

Kohn, L. D. (1978) "Relationships in the Structure and Function of Receptors from Glycoprotein Hormones, Bacterial Toxins and Interferon", in *Receptors and Recognition* Series **A5**, (ed. Cuatrecasas, P. and Greaves, M. F.) Chapman & Hall, London, 133–212.

Lerner, R. A. and Bergsma, D. (eds.) (1978) *The Molecular Basis of Cell–Cell Interaction*, Alan Liss, New York. (Reviews).

Poste, G. and Nicolson, G. L. (eds.) (1977) *The Synthesis, Assembly and Turnover of Cell Surface Components*, North-Holland, Amsterdam. (Reviews).

Rauvala, H. and Finne, J. (1979) "Structural Similarity of the Terminal Carbohydrate Sequences of Glycoproteins and Glycolipids", *FEBS Letters*, **97**, 1–8.

Schachter, H. and Tilley, C. A. (1978) "The Biosynthesis of Human Blood Group Substances", *MTP International Rev. Biochem.*, **16**, 209–246.

Staneloni, R. J. and Leloir, L. F. (1979) "The Biosynthetic Pathways of the Asparagine-Linked Oligosaccharides of Glycoproteins", *Trends in Biochem. Sci.*, **4**, 65–67.

Sturgess, J., Moscarello, M. and Schachter, H. (1978) "The Structure and Biosynthesis of Membrane Glycoproteins", *Current Topics Membranes Transport*, **11**, 15–105.

Turco, S. J. and Robbins, P. W. (1979) "The Initial Stages of Processing of Protein-Bound Oligosaccharides *In Vitro*", *J. Biol. Chem.*, **254**, 4560–4567.

Chapter 10

Ashcroft, S. J. H. and Randle, P. J. (1975) "The Pancreas and Insulin Release", in *Diabetes, its Physiological and Biochemical Basis*, (ed. Vallance-Owen, J.) M.T.P. Press, Lancaster, 31–62.

Fain, J. N. (1978) "Hormones, Receptors and Cyclic Nucleotides", in *Receptors and Recognition* Series **A6** (ed. Cuatrecasas, P. and Greaves, M. F.) Chapman & Hall, London, 1–61.

Felig, P., Sherwin, R. S., Soman, V., Wahren, J., Hendler, R., Sacca, L., Eigler, N., Goldberg, D. and Walesky, M. (1979) "Hormonal Interactions in the Regulation of Blood Glucose", *Recent Progress Hormone Research*, **35**, 501–529.

Klacho, D. M., Anderson, R. R. and Heinberg, M. (eds.) (1979) *Hormones and Energy Metabolism*, (Advan. Exp. Med. Biol., **111**). (Reviews).

Malkinson, A. M. (1975) *Hormone Action*, Chapman & Hall, London.

Notkins, A. L. (1979) "The Cause of Diabetes", *Scientific American*, **241**, (5), 56–67.

Pilkis, S. J., Park, C. R. and Claus, T. H. (1978) "Hormonal Control of Hepatic Gluconeogenesis", *Vitamins and Hormones*, **36**, 383–460.

Varner, J. E. (1978) "Mode of Action of Plant Hormones", *MTP International Rev. Biochem.*, **20**, 189–218.

White, A., Handler, P., Smith, E. L., Hill, R. L. and Lehman, I. R. (1978) *Principles of Biochemistry*, 6th edition, McGraw-Hill, New York.

POSTSCRIPT TO BIBLIOGRAPHY

Burman, D., Holton, J. B. and Pennock, C. A. (eds.) (1980) *"Inherited Disorders of Carbohydrate Metabolism"*, MTP Press Ltd., Lancaster, England. (Reviews relevant to Chapters 7 and 10).

Denton, R. M. and Halestrap, A. P. (1979) "Regulation of Pyruvate Metabolism in Mammalian Tissues", *Essays in Biochem.*, **15**, 37–77. (Relevant to Chapters 2 and 3).

Gooday, G. W. and Trinci, A. P. J. (1980) "Wall Structure and Biosynthesis in Fungi", *30th Symp. Soc. Gen. Microbiol.*, 207–251. (Chapter 8).

Hems, D. A. and Whitton, P. D. (1980) "Control of Hepatic Glycogenolysis", *Physiological Reviews*, **60**, 1–50. (Chapters 7 and 10).

Moore, T. C. (1979) *Biochemistry and Physiology of Plant Hormones*, Springer-Verlag, Berlin. (Chapter 10).

Nieto, A. and Castano, J. G. (1980) "Control *in vivo* of Rat Liver Phosphofructokinase by Glucagon and Nutritional Changes", *Biochem. J.* **186**, 953–957. (Chapter 10).

Rodbell, M. (1980) "The Role of Hormone Receptors and GTP-regulatory Proteins in Membrane Transduction", *Nature, Lond.*, **284**, 17–22. (Chapter 10).

Snell, K. (1980) "Muscle Alanine Synthesis and Hepatic Gluconeogenesis", *Biochem. Soc. Trans.*, **8**, 205–213. (Chapter 3).

Stephen, A. M. (1980) "Plant Carbohydrates", *Encyclopedia of Plant Physiology: New Series* Vol **8**, Springer-Verlag, Berlin, 555–584. (Chapter 8).

Svennerholm, L., Mandel, P., Dreyfus, H. and Urban, P. F. (eds.) (1980) *Structure and Function of Gangliosides*, (Advan. Exp. Med. Biol., **125**). (Chapter 9).

Wang, J. H. and Waisman, D. M. (1979) "Calmodulin and its Role in the Second Messenger System", *Current Topics in Cell. Regulation*, **15**, 47–107. (Chapter 10).

INDEX